Praise for *7 Day Chakras*

"A new and refreshing perspective on working with the seven energies of the yogic chakra system. Shai Tubali invites us to see ourselves as chakra personalities living in a time-based system of seven days, each one with a specific chakra influence. Highly recommend this book for self-reflection and living fully in each day, conscious and awake."

—Colette Baron-Reid, intuition expert, author, and
founder of Oracle School®

"Well, what an interesting read! There's always more to know about chakras, and Shai gives an excellent account to deepen your understanding. This book is an absolute joy and practical at the same time, presenting numerous suggestions and meditations to work with daily. He gives fascinating historical information about the chakras, then brings them right up to date, illuminating a path to deep understanding of self and one's soul journey."

—Patricia Mercier, author of
The Chakra Bible and *Chakra Experience*

····· 7 DAY ·····
CHAKRAS

About the Author

Shai Tubali is an international speaker, author, and spiritual teacher. He is one of Europe's leading authorities in the field of chakras and the subtle body, and he has published more than twelve books in Europe and the US. Shai also founded Human Greatness, an international center in Berlin, Germany.

······ 7 DAY ······
CHAKRAS

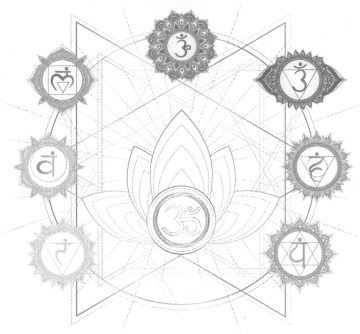

Daily Energy Work to Balance Your Life
SHAI TUBALI

Llewellyn Publications
Woodbury, Minnesota

FIRST EDITION
Second Printing, 2022

Book design by Samantha Peterson
Cover design by Kevin R. Brown
Chakra figure on page 29 by Mary Ann Zapalac

Llewellyn Publications is a registered trademark of Llewellyn Worldwide Ltd.

Library of Congress Cataloging-in-Publication Data
Names: Tubali, Shai (Writer on self-actualization), author.
Title: 7 day chakras : daily energy work to balance your life / Shai
   Tubali.
Other titles: Seven day chakras
Description: First edition. | Woodbury, Minnesota : Llewellyn Publications,
   [2021] | Includes bibliographical references. | Summary: "An
   easy-to-use, step-by-step practice that shows you how to integrate
   chakra energy work into your daily lifestyle" —Provided by publisher.
Identifiers: LCCN 2020058334 (print) | LCCN 2020058335 (ebook) | ISBN
   9780738766928 (paperback) | ISBN 9780738767017 (ebook)
Subjects: LCSH: Chakras.
Classification: LCC BF1442.C53 T828 2021 (print) | LCC BF1442.C53 (ebook)
   | DDC 294.5/43—dc23
LC record available at https://lccn.loc.gov/2020058334
LC ebook record available at https://lccn.loc.gov/2020058335

Llewellyn Publications
A Division of Llewellyn Worldwide Ltd.
2143 Wooddale Drive
Woodbury, MN 55125-2989
www.llewellyn.com

Printed in the United States of America

Other Books by Shai Tubali

CONTENTS

DISCLAIMER

This book is not intended to provide medical or mental health advice nor to take the place of advice and treatment from your primary care provider. Always consult your doctor or another qualified healthcare professional before beginning any dietary regimen. Neither the publisher nor the author take any responsibility for any possible consequences from any treatment to any person reading or following the information in this book.

INTRODUCTION

When the chakras were discovered over two thousand years ago in ancient India, they were initially recognized as powerful energy centers that could be activated through visualizations and mantras. Over time, the concept of these seven inner forces has been greatly developed by numerous seers and experts of the subtle body. Nowadays, it is quite common for the chakras to be considered a comprehensive system that profoundly impacts all levels of our being, including physical health, emotional development, mental balance, and meditative potential. In fact, the more researchers and scholars look into the chakras, the more we realize that they provide us with the most holistic internal map to navigate our psychological and spiritual realms.

In my own two-decade research into the chakra system—which has been inspired by direct investigation, traditional initiations, ancient and modern literature, and chakra work with thousands of people—I have come to appreciate the chakras as the elements through which people communicate with life's different dimensions. I think of them as seven types of experiences, perspectives, and intelligences that enable humanity to come into contact with life as a whole.

This insight—that the composition of seven chakras represents the seven dimensions of life—is what brought me to develop the seven-day chakra path. I realized that as soon as we link each consecutive chakra to its corresponding day—transforming Monday into the root chakra day, Tuesday into the sacral chakra day, and so on—we achieve a highly systematic and complete chakra practice as well as a fully realized experience of the week.

The benefits are many. Let me briefly explain the seven-day chakra cycle's two main gifts.

The Ultimate Chakra Practice

This is a whole new level of chakra work that goes far beyond the usual sets of visualizations, mantras, and yoga postures. Whether you are a chakra enthusiast aspiring to turn your passion for chakras into a practical and livable path or you are a beginner who wishes to be introduced to the chakra world, this all-inclusive practice gives structure to all your chakra processes and allows you to easily explore the many possibilities through which you can bring these energy centers to life.

The path is simple: every week you climb the chakra ladder in its entirety, focusing each day on one of the seven steps to energize and empower a specific center. By the time you have reached the end of the week, all seven chakras will be enkindled, and as a result, your inner being becomes luminous from base to crown. This is a weekly practice that you can return to again and again. In fact, the more you repeat it, the more effective it becomes! As you continue to explore the chakras, illumination grows and your journey of self-development accelerates. The chakras become increasingly more balanced, conscious, and unified.

If you are interested in spiritual enlightenment, such a repeated linear activation of all chakras awakens the subtle central column around which these energy centers are entwined. This awakening can greatly support the process that finally leads to the sublime state of mystical unity: unity within yourself and with the totality of existence.

As you systematically devote your entire attention to each of the chakras, you will become aware of your stronger and weaker chakras. You will then be able to enhance the activity of the chakras you recognize as weaker on their designated days. You will feel encouraged to dedicate time and energy to much-needed healing processes, either physical or emotional, that can mend the unbalanced center. And you will realize that in the process of balancing, dormant capacities and qualities that are currently unavailable to you will emerge from the awakening chakra.

An optimal function of a specific chakra promotes physical well-being and emotional balance. Active chakras better absorb and conduct vital life force and efficiently distribute it to their surrounding glands, nerve plexuses, and organs. This enhanced life force works to unblock clogged energetic regions, and as a result, it expels unwanted emotional and mental excesses. To make use of these healing properties, you may choose to devote the first phase of the weekly cycles to those practices and exercises that heal and balance untreated areas of body and mind, including psychosomatic disorders. The very flow of the chakra week naturally brings attention to different parts of you that have been overlooked because it takes you on a complete journey *through* your body, from your feet through the top of your head.

An Integrative Path That Embraces Life as a Whole

Take a moment to reflect on the current experience of your week by asking yourself the following questions:

1. How do I feel when I plan my week ahead of time?
2. How do I feel at the beginning and the end of the week?
3. Do I give most of my attention to only one or two aspects of my life? If so, what are they?
4. What aspects of my life and my being seem to be neglected or deprioritized?
5. By the end of the week, do I generally feel that I have achieved all that I was hoping for?

Perhaps the most fundamental problem of time management in a stressful Western lifestyle is the feeling that we are chasing our own tails by striving to succeed in many—sometimes contradictory—aspects of our lives. Either we end up over-focused on one or two areas while neglecting all others, or we remain so scattered that very little is actually fulfilled. The seven-day chakra path responds to a deep need for an integrative lifestyle that can masterfully handle reality's demands. As soon as you assign a day to each aspect of your life, you are free from the impossible effort to do everything at once. At the same time, you will begin to notice those aspects that starve for cultivation.

Every week of your life can be a full awakening of body, mind, and spirit. Various traditional paths often advise repeating one particular practice or exercise daily; in this book, the over-concentrated approach is abandoned in favor of practices and activities that are suited for their own specific day. With the wisdom of the chakras, your week turns into a rich and multi-colored journey that starts with the more earthly, physical, and foundational aspects; progresses to emotional, interactive, and social aspects; and ends with the intellectual and spiritual dimensions of your being. With the completion of each cycle, you will feel that you have managed to water all the different flowers of your life's garden. On such a path, everything becomes relevant, meaningful, and equally spiritual, an inseparable part of a greater whole.

Such an integrative path also serves as a powerful self-coaching tool. It first trains you to be grounded. The seven-day chakra path allows you to leave behind your overwhelmed and disorganized vision of life and the oppressive sense of never having enough time. Instead, you are able to take your schedule in your own hands and to focus your energy and attention, fitting the right tasks and events into their ideal times of the week and finding that time is far more pliable and generous than you ever imagined. It is much easier to think of your life in clear categories rather than an indistinguishable cluster of duties and distractions. This path also coaches you by helping you realize more of your wishes and plans, which may have been suppressed in the course of time. In this way, it can show you how to reveal and fulfill much more of your life's potential.

But the seven-day chakra path is not just about effectively handling your time and various missions. This system brings the sense that you can create your schedule and, as a result, your own being and life. Time is not a measuring tool; it is a creative opportunity, a field of possibilities, like an empty canvas on which you can draw your life.

Your tools of creation are not some borrowed concept, religious or other. Chakras live deep inside you as intuitive guiding forces that lead you to complete self-creation and mastery over life's different aspects. Thus, they are the ideal way to regain the sense that the week's cycle is potentially a journey of creation. In this book, the practices and activities suggested for each day are only inspiring ideas to get you started; as soon as you grasp the underlying principles, you can become your own creator and design the experiences of your days.

As a part of this act of creation, you begin to imbue each day with intention. *You* give the day its meaning by coloring it with the unique color of the chakra. Your days are no longer Monday or Tuesday, but the Day of Grounding and the Day of Joy. Because time is an empty canvas, most people are just carried away by an unintentional and coincidental flow of events, randomly experiencing whatever comes their way. With this path, you become proactive, initiating life's experiences, thus shifting from powerlessness to co-creation.

Obviously, the chakra days are not some cosmic frequencies that you are tuning in to. After all, you will probably arrange your very own seven-day cycle around the conventional time frame of the culture you live in, starting the cycle on Saturday, Sunday, or Monday. Your week is therefore empowered by your own intention, bringing to life the inner clock of your subtle body. However, for those of you who appreciate shamanic rituals, natural cycles, and sacred lifestyles, it will feel like tuning in to a larger cosmic intelligence which endows both the week and the day with an exceptional ambience.

Some of us long for a sacred touch in our hyper-secularized life, a connection to a context greater than ourselves. Since chakras can be understood as seven universal rays of the cosmic sun, their presence in your life as an ongoing daily path can fulfill this longing. As you journey each week from the mundane to the spiritual and then descend once again, empowered by spiritual forces, you become filled with this sense of a sacred cycle. Many claim that they do not like rituals, yet our current lifestyle has become quite ritualistic in its endless repetition mixed with a pressing feeling of rushing forward and going nowhere. This seven-day chakra path is an opportunity to feel both the healthy cycle of the week and a steady and authentic process of growth. Tuning in to the chakra cycle can be highly attractive to children as well, who rejoice in having more imaginative references for the different days of the week.

How to Use This Book

In the main chapters of this book, we will delve into the unique adventure of each of the seven chakra days. Each day will be introduced with its individual essence and energy, specific type of happiness and meaning, gifts and powers of healing and balance, affirmations, activities, practices, and challenges. Before we get to that, here are some important guidelines on ways to integrate the seven-day chakra path into your life.

The Importance of the Morning Practice

The morning practice is the most crucial time of your chakra day. Through his 2018 book *The 5 AM Club*, leadership expert Robin Sharma has become an ardent promoter of the concept of early rising as a way to maximize one's achievements, health, and focus. According to Sharma, the first part of the day is also the most crucial. Waking up as early as possible, while everyone else is still asleep, implies zero distractions and is therefore an ideal time to expand productivity and creativity. More specifically, he treats 5:00 to 6:00 a.m. as the "victory hour," recommending it be divided into three twenty-minute parts, starting with strong physical exercise, moving to a reflection on the day's goals and vision, and culminating in studying something new. In a lifestyle where there is never enough time, this prescription identifies an oasis of focus.

In the context of the seven-day chakra path, the morning practice is just as essential. By beginning your practice immediately upon waking, you are giving shape to the entire day; you brush it with the colors of the chakra and release its energies and powers into the rest of the day. You do not necessarily have to wake up at 5:00 a.m., but if possible, get used to waking up one hour before your duties and routine take over. Nowadays, people are flooded with information and technological interaction that expect us to always be available and efficient, so resist that temptation and start practicing before you open the gates of your mind to the world. Wake up to a silent, untouched day, a day that is for you to create—*your* day.

The seven-day chakra path is not as focused on maximizing productivity as Sharma's approach—actually, there are four days in this book that recommend doing the very opposite! Within each chapter you will find a detailed description of the recommended morning practice for each chakra day, but the structure is identical: take at least one hour for the practice, which ideally contains three consecutive stages (as with Sharma's concept, the hour can be conveniently divided into three twenty-minute parts):

Activation. Select any type of chakra activation; there will be options among the suggested practices of the individual chapters. I recommend activating the chakra by applying its corresponding section from either the Smiling into Your Chakras meditation or the Chakra Flowering meditation (found in chapter 3). Some prefer to be more physical and dynamic during their activation and choose to dance, paint, do yoga postures or breathing exercises, or any form of dynamic meditation. The point is to select whatever method of activation seems to stimulate the chakra according to its chapter's description. Truly, the very act of turning your attention to the chakra stimulates it. While activating, repeat one of the suggested affirmations like a mantra. Make use of the provided affirmations (or your own) throughout the day by writing them on sticky notes attached to your computer, desk, wallet, or water bottle, or simply let them echo in your mind.

Inspiration. Enrich yourself by learning something that best represents and expresses the energies and capacities that you wish to awaken in yourself during this chakra day—first and foremost, you are learning in order to evoke your own motivation and excitement. Ideally, prepare your source of inspiration beforehand (creative days such as Tuesday, the Day of Joy, and Friday, the Day of Expression, are most suitable for gathering such materials). There are plenty of recommended pathways of inspiration within the chapters, but the more you open up, the more you will be amazed at the countless videos, books, speeches, and films that can ignite your focus.

Vision. Dedicate some time to journal about how exactly you are going to respond to the day's chakra frequency. How will you live this day fully? Close your eyes and, in as much detail as possible, envision yourself in a state of ideal and undisturbed embodiment of the chakra's energy. See yourself in real-life situations, successfully responding to the challenges of this chakra. Perhaps you want to see yourself responding to certain challenges that you are expecting on this day. How would you respond to challenges using the day's frequency? Are there some blockages that might hinder your capacity to fulfill it? If they feel insurmountable, perhaps your day should be devoted to facing them.

At the end of the vision stage, choose one activity and one practice as your minimum commitment to the chakra day. Activities (under the title "Engage Your ___ Chakra") are actions in life, and practices (titled "Practices to Empower Your Day") are internal techniques and meditations. These, combined with the morning practice, are enough to enjoy a fully realized day. If an activity or practice can take place during the last hour before you go to sleep, that creates a perfect circle, holding the day from both ends and enabling you to separate from its energy with one last focus.

Pay Attention to the Structure of the Week

Monday, most commonly thought of as the first day of the week, is the time to thoughtfully consider all the things you want to accomplish throughout the week in the different fields of life. This is not just about work plans, tasks, and meetings; it is an opportunity to define what you hope to accomplish this week as an integrated and multilayered human being. At what point in your development do you wish to find yourself by the end of the week? This may include your food habits, gaining a profound understanding of meditation, attaining a deeper creativity, or creating a more balanced relationship with your body. As part of your Monday assessment, make sure to include all that you have accomplished in the previous week in order to appreciate the gradual process of building your life.

The chakra cycle recommends three days as the most fiery and intense ones: Monday (root chakra day, or the Day of Grounding); Wednesday (solar plexus chakra day, or the Day of Power), and Friday (throat chakra day, or the Day of Expression). These are the best days to make important decisions, define goals and ambitions, and push yourself a little more. For those of you who are overactive, there will be enough opportunities to cool down during the week. For those who are more passive, these are the days that urge you to remember to prioritize your higher dreams and visions. It is highly balancing—and quite different from the Western tradition of perpetual work and stress—to acknowledge the fact that the chakras offer three days of action and four that cultivate less "productive" values, such as joy, emotion, intellect, and spirit.

As you begin the seven-day chakra cycle, you will quickly identify that some days come naturally to you; indeed, in so many ways you are probably already practicing that day's lessons. Realize that your stronger days can be deepened and further explored as well; do not assume that you already know and live all the possible depths of a chakra.

It is likely that you will want to start a long-term project on one of the days. For example, writing parts of a book every Tuesday and Friday or researching a certain field every Saturday (the Day of Wisdom). Starting a long-term practice is a good choice because it mixes changing practices and ongoing activities. The changing practices keep your progression from one cycle to another refreshed and surprising, while ongoing projects employ the path's potential to bring your ideas and visions to a full manifestation.

You can even take it a step further and set up special events, such as celebrations or meetings, on their ideal days. However, be cautious not to become over-religious about this concept, insisting on fitting each and every event into your chakra schedule. Some practitioners are perfectionists or tend to exercise total control over their life, so they might become quite agitated when a friend invites them to a birthday party on Monday, the Day of Grounding, or their partner wants to watch a comedy with them on Wednesday, the Day of Power. Use the week's structure as a platform to play on while orienting yourself to the general spirit of the day. This is why the morning practice is so significant: the day itself is far more susceptible to pressures and expectations.

That said, even within the ordinary flow of events, you can implement the day's perspective and energy, using the lens of the chakra to look at whatever you do. Your work is a good example; it probably expresses the qualities of only one or two chakras, the chakras that are naturally your strongest. But the work itself can be viewed from different angles and carry a different flavor on certain days—and often, such unusual perspectives can help you to better cope with challenges at work.

Generally, there is no need to immerse yourself in the chakra frequency all day long. Do not be troubled if you forget all about your chakra focus for several hours. Some days require dealing with burdensome matters that inevitably occupy your attention. Early morning and night practices can ensure that the energy of the day is retained even on such all-consuming days.

Lastly, if you wish to be supported on your seven-day chakra path, you are invited to subscribe to my online campus and community: https://activespirits.net/en/. This platform is dedicated to sharing inspiring quotes, videos, audios, meditations, chakra activations, and elaborate courses on a daily basis. These will enhance and unfold the different chakra days. If you choose to involve yourself in this community, you will also be able to exchange ideas and materials with members to enrich each other's path.

Small Steps for a Big Path

Some will find it easy to reorient their life swiftly and effectively according to the seven-day chakra principles. Others may experience this adaptation as a struggle, establishing an unnatural routine while facing the strong opposition of their own drives and an unsupportive environment. If you belong to the latter, there are practical ways in which you can easily but firmly ground yourself in this empowering way of life.

The key here is forming habits. Only habits—automatic patterns of behavior—can enable you to make the shift from struggling to maintain this lifestyle to embracing an effortless way of being. If you can make the chakra week something that your unconscious mind supports, you avoid the obvious pitfall of relying solely on belief and effort. Ideally, the chakra week is much like a thoughtless pattern.

This does not mean that the cycle does not involve heightened awareness and expanded consciousness as a result of the ongoing activation of the seven chakras, but you are not expected to concentrate really hard every morning to invoke the day's energy. You should feel that the day draws you into it, that it somehow exists prior to your conscious attention and that you are naturally inclined to participate in it. This will enable you to delve more deeply into the potential empowerment and insight of each day while relying on the unchanging, solid foundations of your new habit.

The following one-hour writing practice could be a significant first step:

1. Devote twenty minutes to answering these two questions: What are the lasting changes that I wish to create in my life? Are there some unfulfilled, or seemingly unfulfillable, changes that I have despaired of considering? Use this time to take a broad look at all the different aspects of your life and being.

2. Next, dedicate twenty minutes to journaling about habitual changes: What old habits do I want to discard? What new habits do I want to establish?

3. During the remaining twenty minutes, divide your habits according to the categories of the seven chakra days: grounding, joy, power, love, expression, wisdom, and spirit. Specify the actions that need to be repeated to bring your old habits to an end and to form the desired habits. This simple process will help you to shift from abstract concepts and vague intentions to the most practical vision of your new life.

Think of your weekly habits as effective channels that enable the big changes you have always hoped for to effortlessly flow into your life. The big change we are talking about is, of course, aligning your life with the chakra cycle. If this way of life becomes a habit for you, you will never need to discipline yourself to live by this principle. For this to happen, you should first create the cues that are powerful enough to make you unintentionally respond with the right mindset and action.

Here are fourteen cues that can serve as signposts throughout the week. You don't have to follow all of them to jump-start the chakra-week engine. You can also add more personal cues that orient you even more immediately and efficiently.

1. At the beginning of each week—or, even better, at the beginning of each month—set up events suitable for the relevant days. Ideally, they should involve and depend on others. Events that can be repeated every week are best, like a new tradition. For instance, dancing with friends every Tuesday (the Day of Joy) or having a romantic dinner with your partner every Thursday (the Day of Love). Repeated events that involve others will keep you naturally close to the heartbeat of the chakra week.

2. Buy a beautiful yearly planner and enjoy preparing your entire year—or what is left of it—with titles and colors for each day of the week. To speed up the process, you can also design and print seven stickers. With this simple technique, you will receive a reminder of your new lifestyle every time you open your diary.

3. When planning your week ahead, reserve a one-hour slot in your daily schedule. Avoid the temptation to insert

activities in these slots. This availability can encourage you to focus on the chakra day during these times.

4. At the beginning of the week, or the night before the next chakra day, create signs with visual or verbal reminders and spread them in noticeable places. An important sign could be placed in the spot that is the first thing you see when you wake up. The good thing about these images and quotes is that you don't need to create new ones every day—they will be relevant fifty-two times a year!

5. Schedule messages and reminders, via your email account or your cell phone, that will be sent to you as quick attention enhancers on an hourly basis, or perhaps twice a day. For example, a text message on Tuesday, the Day of Joy, could be "Don't forget to smile!"

6. Every night, prepare an inspiring video that will wait in an open window on your computer until the next morning. Make sure that you create seven separate files to classify any powerful video you may encounter in order to avoid starting all over again every week.

7. Before going to sleep, position unavoidable objects that will serve as strong reminders of the chakra day. For example, place your meditation chair at the center of the living room, or prepare an outfit that expresses, in either color or style, the next chakra day.

8. At night, set up an exciting environment for the next day. This can be as simple as arranging a fruit or vegetable bowl that conveys (in color or energy) the chakra day. There are a great variety of chakra products—incense,

cups, candles, and music—that can be used for their relevant day.

9. Every morning, read the section "Feel the Day" in the relevant chapter. This section is specifically designed to help you tune in to the day's vibration. When you feel the day rather than hold it in your mind as a concept, it is far more difficult to forget about it.

10. Encourage an open-minded friend to follow the seven-day chakra path with you. Don't force it on anyone—offer it and let them decide if they want to give it a try, even for a limited period of time. If you do find such a willing friend, this can be an enormous support, especially during the first two months when the habit is gradually forming. Send text messages to one another—perhaps "May you have a heart-opening Day of Love" on Thursday —and see if you can practice together or engage in relevant activities. If you have a long-distance friendship, you could always practice or engage through video or on the phone.

11. Use your Facebook or Instagram account to publish posts that are relevant to each day. You don't need to directly dedicate your texts and photos to the day; you could refer to it at the beginning or closing lines of your post (for example, "Since today, according to the chakra week, is the third eye chakra day, or the Day of Wisdom ..."). Synchronizing your posts with the chakra days can create a powerful context: by publicly announcing it on a daily basis and engaging others, even subtly, with this concept, the path may rapidly turn into an effortless habit.

12. Invent small rituals that can be repeated in exactly the same manner, such as making a brief daily prayer as soon as you wake up to concentrate your intention and attention, or separating from the chakra day and feeling the next one using gestures or words just before you fall asleep.

13. Choose to embark on this path by first repeating only one day which seems the easiest to you, either because this day is technically the most available one or because it is in harmony with your chakra personality type. (We'll talk more about this in chapter 3.) As soon as this day has become habituated, your entire week will revolve around it, and it will be easier to add the other days, one after the other.

14. Be a part of a vibrant community that is composed of people who follow the chakra week. As I already mentioned, my online learning platform is arranged around this concept to enable its participants this kind of complete self-fulfillment. Upon registration, you will start receiving a daily email that will provide you with the right chakra orientation and direct you to new uploaded content such as lectures, guided meditations, and courses. In addition, you will be able to interact with other learners and enkindle each other's enthusiasm and understanding. If you follow the path all by yourself, such an external framework could be crucial in making this path an unshakable habit that bears long-lasting results.

Luckily, the seven-day chakra path also grants you immediate rewards, not just long-term ones that will begin to show after sufficient repetition. This, in itself, is a crucial factor in habit formation.[1] Rewarding feelings, as well as instant results, are going to permeate the experience of the day and the week. Gratifying states of mind and body will be experienced at the end of every week, but also at the end of every day and at the end of every small gesture that you make toward the day. When your chakras, the seven wheels of energy, spin more quickly in response to your conscious attention, they immediately begin to emit new levels of awareness, inner wholeness, and peace. What could be more rewarding than that?

---

1   Wood, *Good Habits*, 116–17.

EXPLORING THE CHAKRAS AND THE WEEK

This book is all about a marriage of two ancient traditions: the seven-day week and the chakra system; two traditions which, perhaps, were meant to be together.

The first tradition, the seven-day week cycle, began around 2,600 years ago, yet it is fervently followed to this day: six days of labor and one day of rest. This concept, which is neither natural nor obvious, originates from Judaism, which brought to life a six-day cycle culminating in the Sabbath. During the second century BCE, the astrological seven-day cycle, synchronized with seven planets, was independently developed, with Saturday as the first day of its week. We owe the most prevailing seven-day cycle (that of Monday to Sunday) to the church, which combined the Jewish and astrological weeks while transforming, for religious and political reasons, the first day of the Jewish week—Sunday—into its very own "peak" day.[2]

The second tradition, the chakra system, also emerged around 2,600 years ago, mentioned for the first time in the Hindu Upanishads and 400 years later in the Yoga Sutras of Patanjali.[3] These early signs of the theory of the subtle body and its energy centers, or psychic centers of consciousness, particularly thrived in the later tradition of Tantric Yoga during the second half of the first millennium. There were many chakra systems back then—ranging from a more modest system of five chakras all the way to twenty-one—but somewhere around the fifteenth century, the seven-chakra system became the dominant one. With the help of the orientalist John Woodroffe and some occultists, this system has become the version accepted by the Western world and modernized as a ladder of psychological development.[4]

By now I hope you have traced the common ground of these two traditions: the cycle of seven. This shared underlying principle seems to wed the seven days and the seven chakras quite effortlessly: seven days for seven chakras and the other way around.

But before rushing to the wedding, let us take a deeper look at the basics of the chakra system.

What Are Chakras?

The earliest known reference to the chakras in the documented history of ancient India is this quote:

---

2   Zerubavel, *Seven Day Circle*, 8, 14.

3   Judith, "History of the Chakra System."

4   Wallis, "Real Story on the Chakras."

> [Some] have seen [the Lord of Love] riding in wis-
> dom on his chariot, with seven colors as horses
> and six wheels to represent the whirling spokes of
> time.[5]

The quote is completely metaphorical: the true self within us rides on its chariot with seven colors as horses and six wheels. But what is the chariot that it rides in wisdom?

Chakras are part of a greater discovery made by the ancient seers of India. More than 2,500 years ago, they came to realize that each of us has two bodies. The first is the easily perceived physical body and the second is the subtle or energy body—our true self's chariot. While each of our bodies has its own anatomy and physiology, the two are deeply intertwined and even share some common characteristics.

The subtle body consists of thousands of flexible and hollow tubes that the ancients called *nadis* (literally, "a flow"). As a matter of fact, the Tantric scriptures suggest that this highly complex network contains no less than 72,000 nadis! This network can be compared to our physical nervous system, but its function is extremely different: nadis conduct subtle energies and forces, such as *prana* (vital force), that sustain and enable our mental and spiritual existence.

Fortunately, we are not expected to be aware of the entire network. Within this complex structure, only three are truly crucial, since they control the flow of prana and consciousness in all the other nadis as well as the awakening of our spiritual consciousness: the central channel (or *sushumna*) and the two side channels (called *pingala* and *ida*), which are entwined around it in

---

5   Easwaran, *The Upanishads*, 227.

a serpentine movement. The straight central channel runs close to the front side of the spine and is in fact considered to be the energetic spine that holds the entire structure of our subtle body. Like streams that diverge from a great river and return to merge in it, the two side channels have six convergence points along the central channel. In these exact points, the first six chakras reside.

The chakras are smaller channels that branch off at various points along the central channel to form channel wheels or vortices (*chakra* literally translates to "wheel"). Add to that the fact that the three main channels converge in six of these power points and you will understand why chakras are considered to be major junctions of energy. How many chakras there are depends on your choice to treat two or more of these energy centers as just one center or to split some of them into subcenters. This is the reason for the diverse chakra systems that sometimes consist of five, six, eight, or even twenty-one chakras. However, the division that has become most acceptable is the seven-chakra system, and the reasons for this will be explained in the last section of this chapter. The specific locations of the chakras also vary, depending on the tradition, although they are never dramatically different. Often the chakra's precise location is selected by the tradition to lead its students to certain results.

Common Chakra Misunderstandings

There are two important misunderstandings about the chakras' locations and characteristics. First, it is commonly believed that chakras reside in the front part of the body, close to the skin. It is true that this is the most immediate way they can be felt, but in reality, these are only the chakras' contact centers or trigger points, called *kshetram*. These contact points are significant, since they are also the chakras' interaction with the outer world, and they are therefore the layer that most strongly experiences any emotionally provoking situations or other external pressures. The true location of the chakras, however, is inside the central channel, the sushumna, close to the frontal side of the spine. When meditating on a chakra, it is therefore most effective and powerful to move with your attention from the frontal part to the center of your body and to contact the chakra's power there.

A second source of confusion is the widespread belief that chakras have certain colors and shapes. Many try to identify the color green inside their heart chakra or the color purple in their third eye chakra. And the confusion grows because different traditions suggest different colors to focus on! The reason for this difference is simple: each tradition inserts certain visualizations, mantras, syllables, or colors into these energy centers with the intention to enhance the chakra's activity, awaken its dormant powers, or release its subtle layer of consciousness for the sake of spiritual development. This means that the known approach that correlates the seven chakras with the seven colors of the rainbow is purely metaphorical.

It is beautiful to liken the chakra system to the way white light breaks through a prism into seven colors, but do not be disappointed when you are failing to find these colors inside your chakras. In this book, I will offer using the rainbow colors and what are traditionally called "seed sounds" to enhance your daily chakra practice, but remember that these are just methods, not descriptions. The seed sounds ("Beeja mantras"), which come from the world of Tantric Hinduism, are vibrations created through voice: each of the seven sounds is applied to stimulate a particular chakra.

The Role of Chakras

Chakras are not just mechanical conductors and regulators of subtle energies. What actually makes them so important is the fact that they act as centers of interchange between the physical, energetic, emotional, mental, and spiritual layers of our being. Chakras create contact points between these dimensions and enable the passage of energy from one dimension to another.

For instance, chakras possess the ability to transform subtle energies into physical energies and the other way around. This unique position in the meeting point of the physical body and the subtle body makes each chakra a highly influential factor in the health of the glands, nerve plexuses, and organs that surround it. But, at the same time, nutritional choices and lifestyle can enhance or hinder the activity of the chakras. Similarly, the unique position of the chakras in the meeting point of the energetic dimension and the emotional and mental dimensions makes these energy vortices deeply associated with the condition of our psyche. This means that your chakras are affected by the degree of your emotional and mental balance and that they carry within them psychological impressions and imprints. On the other hand, the way a certain chakra functions greatly determines aspects of your emotional and mental well-being: an optimally active chakra instantly reduces the chatter of the mind, calms down emotional turmoil, and induces positive qualities and behaviors.

If you wish to initiate direct contact with your chakras, try one of these quick experiments. First, close your eyes for ten minutes and visualize a central channel piercing the center of your body from the perineum all the way up to the top of the center of your head. Then, simply look for power points along this channel; the more energetically loaded areas, where you feel a greater intensity or vibration, are most likely the chakras. If you wish to be even more thorough in this experiment, take five more minutes and try to sense the kshetram, the frontal part of the chakras, by scanning the front of your body from the upper forehead all the way down to the point below the genitals. Can you identify areas that are more active than others? Compare the results of the first and second examinations. If areas within the central channel correspond to areas at the front line, these are definitely chakras.

The second experiment can enable you to identify the subtle connections that specific chakras have with emotional issues. Close your eyes for ten minutes and start your meditation by thinking about a significant emotional conflict you have experienced lately or a current challenge in your life. You can even bring up an unresolved issue from your past—if it has not been fully resolved, it is still somewhere inside your body. After at least five minutes of contemplation, look for the area in your body that responds to the issue. That area is most likely a chakra, since the conflict is not really in your physical body but rather within the subtle body. As far as we know, nobody has a physically broken heart—the broken heart is an experience of the heart chakra!

The fact that chakras exist on the border that connects all the different layers of our being is the source of their tremendous relevance to processes of physical and psychosomatic healing, emotional and mental balancing, and spiritual enlightenment. Each of the seven chakras can function on four levels:

- Dysfunctional: minimal activity, deeply blocked
- Functional: a moderate degree of flow

- Balanced: harmonious flow
- Awakened: pure and refined energy flow

You can develop the chakra function in one of the two ways: the direct, traditional path (working on the chakras directly through energetic purification) or the indirect path, which focuses on responding to the psychological and spiritual issues that are related to each of the chakras. Any trauma work you do and any meditation you practice alters—either temporarily or irreversibly, depending on the depth of the transformative impact—the condition of the relevant chakra.

Each of the seven chakras represents particular aspects of your subtle body, psyche, and spiritual consciousness. In this sense, chakras are quite linear and vertical, like a ladder of development that starts with the most earthly level of existence and culminates in the most spiritual. When you sincerely respond to the psychological challenges and issues of one chakra, you bring one level of your being to balance and can then climb another step on your inner ladder. This vertical nature of the chakras has made them one of the most effective and easy-to-understand internal roadmaps. With their help, you can navigate your psychological evolution and attain a holistic emotional maturity or follow your spiritual evolution all the way to its final fulfillment in the seventh, uppermost crown chakra.

The Seven Chakras

Here is a brief overview of each of the seven chakra's most fundamental characteristics.

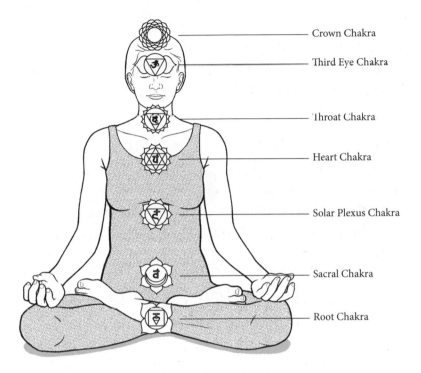

Crown Chakra

Third Eye Chakra

Throat Chakra

Heart Chakra

Solar Plexus Chakra

Sacral Chakra

Root Chakra

Root Chakra

Traditional Name: Muladhara

Location: Slightly inside the perineum (kshetram: none)

Element: Earth

Associated Color: Red

Seed Mantra: Lam

Day of the Week: Monday

Psychological Aspect: Instinct, earthly and biological existence, security, groundedness, physical foundation and health, fear of instability and change, trauma

Sacral Chakra

Traditional Name: Swadhisthana

Location: Base of the spinal column, at the level of the coccyx or tailbone (kshetram: at the level of the pubic bone)

Element: Water

Associated Color: Orange

Seed Mantra: Vam

Day of the Week: Tuesday

Psychological Aspect: Feeling and impulse, vitality, adventure, totality, enjoyment, sensuality, pursuit of pleasure, sexuality, shame, the unconscious

Solar Plexus Chakra

Traditional Name: Manipura

Location: Behind the navel (kshetram: at the navel); anatomically related to the solar plexus

Element: Fire

Associated Color: Yellow

Seed Mantra: Ram

Day of the Week: Wednesday

Psychological Aspect: Will, individuality, independence, ambition, intensity, courage, control, anger

Heart Chakra

Traditional Name: Anahata

Location: Behind the center of the chest, midway between the two breasts (kshetram: center of the chest)

Element: Air

Associated Color: Green

Seed Mantra: Yam

Day of the Week: Thursday

Psychological Aspect: Emotions, relationships, love, attachment and dependency, betrayal and disappointment, forgiveness, letting go

Throat Chakra

Traditional Name: Vishuddhi

Location: Behind the throat pit (kshetram: front of the neck, at the throat pit)

Element: Ether

Associated Color: Blue

Seed Mantra: Ham

Day of the Week: Friday

Psychological Aspect: Communication, self-expression, leadership, manifestation, vision, authenticity, transparency

Third Eye Chakra

Traditional Name: Ajna

Location: Behind the eyebrow center (kshetram: mid-eyebrow center)

Element: Light

Associated Color: Purple

Seed Mantra: Om

Day of the Week: Saturday

Psychological Aspect: Intellect, clarity, insight, mental order, discrimination, attention, curiosity

Crown Chakra

Traditional Name: Sahasrara

Location: Center of the top of the head, in the brain (kshetram: none)

Element: Cosmos; pure light and source of creation

Associated Color: Violet and white

Seed Mantra: Ah

Day of the Week: Sunday

Psychological Aspect: Spirit, meditation, transcendence, timelessness, nonattachment, divine nature, universality

• • • • •

Since chakras are influenced both directly and indirectly, the seven-day chakra path embraces a multilevel approach in order to fully awaken each of the seven chakras. The activities and practices—including affirmations and mantras, meditations, psychological processes, and facing relevant challenges—activate the chakras energetically, emotionally, mentally, and spiritually. Together, the activities and practices bring the chakras—and as a result, life as a whole—into perfect harmony.

The Seven-Day Week and the Chakras

Our entire experience of life is based on the passage from one week to another—a fixed, unchanging cycle of seven twenty-four-hour days that has been accepted as an inherent cornerstone of everyday life. The sociologist Pitirim Sorokin writes, "We think in week units; we apprehend time in week units ... We live and feel and plan and wish in 'week' terms. It is one of the most important points of 'orientation' in time and social reality."[6] When we wake and immediately recall what day it is, we move from our personal world to participate in the larger rhythm of the world.[7]

Interestingly, the source of this cycle lies in deep spiritual perception and intuition. To begin with, the number seven played a major role in the liturgy, ritual, magic, and art of the ancient civilization of Mesopotamia. The ancient Babylonians even conceived of the universe as a sevenfold entity reigned over by a fusion of seven deities. Soon, seven-day intervals began to symbolically represent the principles of totality and completeness, considered homogenous, closed periods of time.[8]

However, the ancient dwellers of Mesopotamia did not have a real seven-day week. This seems to be a distinctively Jewish contribution to our civilization. Sometime during their exile from the land of Israel, when Jews came into contact with the inhabitants of Mesopotamia and were perhaps somewhat inspired by them, they developed the concept of observing the Sabbath (the seventh day) every seven days. Of course, they had their own story of creation to rely on: according to the Biblical account, it was God himself who first practiced this cycle, with six days of creation followed by a seventh day of divine, refreshing rest. This transformed into one of the Ten Commandments: "Six days shalt thou labour, and do all thy work, but the seventh day is the

---

6   Zerubavel, *Seven Day Circle*, vii.

7   Zerubavel, *Seven Day Circle*, 2–3.

8   Zerubavel, *Seven Day Circle*, 7–8.

Sabbath of the Lord thy God."[9] Accordingly, the Hebrew word *shavúa* (week) is directly related to the word *sheva* (seven), and the word "Sabbath" (Saturday) is translated as: "cease from labor."

Take a quick time leap, nearly 400 years forward, and you will find yet another development of the seven-day cycle, associated with seven planets. At the very heart of the Hellenistic world, Alexandria, astronomers arranged the seven planets in a specific invariable order. Consequently, a successful fusion of astronomy, astrology, and mathematics gave rise to the astrological week, which was seven days long simply because the astronomers happened to identify seven planets.

While the Jewish and astrological weeks evolved quite independently of one another, the happy coincidence of their identical length soon brought them closer—for instance, driving the Jews to finally fix the Sabbath in the "day of Saturn" (Saturday). The astrological week, introduced to the Western world by Rome close to the end of the first century BCE, was eventually merged with the Jewish week by the church that spread the gospel of the seven-day cycle throughout the world. Though the church surrendered to the astrological associations of the seven days, which by then were too widespread to dispense with, it managed to keep Saturday and Sunday as the holy days of the week. Nonetheless, while the early Christians were Jews observing the Sabbath on Saturday, the church, aspiring to distance itself from Judaism, established a separate weekly cycle peaking on Sunday. Following the same logic, Mohammed chose Friday as Islam's peak day.

Perhaps you have noticed from this brief history of the week that it is purely a matter of human invention. Some wrongly believe that the seven-day week derived from the natural lunar

---

9   Exodus 20:8–11 (Authorized King James Version).

cycle. Yet the lunar month cannot be divided into perfect weekly blocks of complete days. Eviatar Zerubavel, a professor of sociology, explains that, unlike the day and the year, our week is an artificial rhythm, intended to "break away from being prisoners of nature and create an artificial world of [our] own."[10] By creating a perfect seven-day week, we control the regularity of human activity and ensure a high-level social organization.

However, the price we pay as individuals is high. The week's purpose is wholly functional, a social and financial engine that enables us to perform tasks regularly and to move in a predictable manner from one week to another. For most of us who lead a secular lifestyle, it is far from an emotional, energetic, or spiritual cycle, completely devoid of its glamorous ancient meaning. It certainly does not feel like tuning in to some balancing rhythm, nor does it encourage the capacity to flow creatively with your time. The general experience of the week is one of wearisome repetition and of rushing forward ceaselessly, with the usual feeling of "Monday blues" as well as the anticipation toward the weekend's release.

José Argüelles, a researcher in the field of art history and aesthetics, identified this problem, claiming that the "artificial timing frequency" has disconnected humanity from the biosphere, moving it entirely to the "technosphere." Convinced that time is the "universal factor of synchronization," he suggested that the experience that people never have enough time and the current cultural convention that "time is money" are both the result of the detachment from humanity's true nature. Instead, he offered a new experience that "time equals art," founded on an alternative

---

10   Zerubavel, *Seven Day Circle*, 4.

calendar which is partly inspired by the Mayan concept of time. Significantly, he too kept the seven-day cycle.[11]

Discontinuing the connection with humanity's calendar may be quite impractical, but perhaps it is time to fill our own experience of the week with deeper content and to place it within a broader context. Here is where the chakra system enters with its miraculous capacity to transform the week forever.

In the same way that there have been other week cycles—like the three ten-day intervals in ancient China and Greece and among the Maori of New Zealand—there have also been other chakra systems. Yet these two traditions, with their mysterious principle of seven, have clearly prevailed. In light of the fact that both initially emerged around the same time, could it be that the week is governed by the very same intuition that has led us to eventually choose the seven-chakra system? It is impressive to note, for instance, that the seven days actually mean 6 + 1—a day of rest separate from the entire week. In the very same way, the seven chakras are 6 + 1, since technically the seventh chakra does not count as a chakra at all. Just like the seventh day, the crown chakra is the resting place. The seventh chakra is the home of Kundalini, where the cycle of growth and evolution no longer takes place.[12]

It is likely that the seven-chakra system has triumphed because of the Babylonians' spiritual intuition that seven represents totality and completeness; this resonates within humanity as a universal code that could aid us in our own completeness. The seven-day cycle *feels* complete, and having seven chakras seems to encompass the entire scope of humanity's qualities, capacities, and challenges.

---

11   Argüelles, "Law of Time."

12   Wallis, "Real Story on the Chakras."

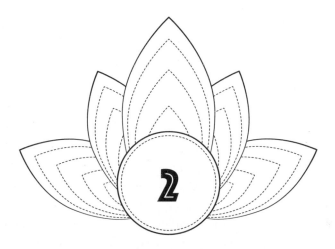

CHAKRAS AND HUMAN NEED

One way of grasping the significance and transformative power of the seven-day chakra path is through the recognition of the variety of human needs.

On the one hand, needs are perhaps the most accessible expression of our chakra psychology. Everyone knows what needs feel like because when they cry for attention inside us, we experience them physically, even when they are emotional or spiritual needs. A need for appreciation, for instance, can make the heart physically ache. On the other hand, the reality of needs is poorly understood, let alone acknowledged and fulfilled.

Too often, people are unable to tell the difference between needs and wants. This distinction is crucial because as long as you treat your needs as wants, you will fail to appreciate how vital they are. After all, wants are a luxury whereas needs are a necessity—something that you *have* to fulfill.

A need is an expression of a certain part of ourselves that is starving. In an ideal state, we function like a good and loving gardener by making sure that we nourish all the different aspects of our being. But when we neglect one or more of these aspects, they appear, sooner or later, in the form of deprivation. Like hunger and thirst—forms of deprivation of two of our most basic needs—when these parts remain unfulfilled, you actually feel thirst and hunger for a certain experience, feeling, or feedback. Think of moments in which you experienced a long, warm hug, a wonderful concert or a deep meditation, and exclaimed, "I really *needed* that!"

This sense of deprivation can appear after a long time if you practice a certain lifestyle that narrowly focuses on the fulfillment of some parts of your being while completely ignoring others. If your day and night are dedicated to climbing the ladder of success, you will tend to overlook—and perhaps even suppress—your need for enjoyment and leisure. As a result, at a certain point in time you will be compelled to meet the pain of deprivation head-on—the realization that this invaluable need has been left behind.

Sometimes, such a life of consistent deprivation causes sudden shifts. This is the law of extremes: if you live in one extreme for long enough, your deprived aspects will accumulate to a degree that they will one day erupt in their most acute and desperate form. Take, for example, businessmen and businesswomen who turn to a spiritual lifestyle overnight or devoutly religious people who suddenly leave everything behind and become intensely secular and indulgent.

When a specific vitamin or mineral is persistently missing from your diet, this chronic shortage will eventually cause symptoms or even disease.[13] In the same way, any need that is consistently ignored in your lifestyle will lead to physical, emotional, mental, or spiritual imbalances. This becomes a deeply revealing fact in light of the understanding that you have more needs than you have ever imagined.

As a human, you are a complex being that consists of many different layers, and each layer has its own needs in order to achieve healthy fulfillment. Here the chakras greatly aid us by comprehensively introducing us to our multilayered being. Chakras function not only as energy centers but also as representations of the different facets of life and existence. They should be thought of as gateways through which we interact with aspects of ourselves and of the world around us. When we activate all seven, we experience life in its totality, from its most material expression to its ultimate spiritual core. We thus manage to become fully realized humans with all the keys of creation in our hands, which we can use to unlock the seven doors of our very own selves. Using the chakras in this way, we can embrace the complexity of our being without missing even one dimension or potential experience. This is what we do in the seven-day chakra path.

As expressions of the seven dimensions of our being, chakras also contain the prescriptions for their optimal functioning: meet their needs for fulfillment and they will become a flourishing energy system that nurtures your body, mind, and spirit. This implies that humans have seven categories of needs. We definitely have more needs than the basic demands for food, water, sleep, or shelter; we also need grounding, joy, power, love, expression,

---

13   Francis, *Never Fear Cancer Again*, 304.

wisdom, and spirit. Those other, more refined needs may not strike you as essentials at first. This is precisely why we push them down, claiming that we do not have enough time for them and that they can wait for one imaginary day when we will suddenly have time.

There are many needs that people disregard as forms of childish neediness that should be overcome. If you do not include all your needs in your to-do list, you will never embark on the journey of total self-fulfillment. But even if you do acknowledge them, the idea of fulfilling all of these needs within the limited framework of a seven-day week may seem insanely unrealistic. Luckily, since the seven-day chakra path centers each day on the fulfillment of one dimension of being, meeting every need becomes an easily achievable task.

Some may argue that the full scope of human needs can only be revealed to us after we have become capable of satisfying the most basic ones. Only then can we recognize that there are other "higher" aspects that are not essentially different from the foundational requirements of a functioning human existence. This, however, is questionable: sometimes, taking care of "luxury" needs can be highly balancing and nourishing; an emotionally satisfying interaction or coming into contact with the beauty of the various arts should not wait until you have fully succeeded in attaining financial stability.

All needs, so the chakras tell us, exist in us simultaneously— and not only as a ladder of increasing refinement. For example, the crown chakra's need for meditation is chronically overlooked by most humans. But as soon as you begin to respond to it, you realize to what extent this has been your *need* for inner peace and quietude rather than your *wish* for spiritual evolution, much like a trace mineral that your body cannot do without.

Maslow's Hierarchy of Human Needs

Abraham Maslow, the father of humanistic psychology, is one of the most cited psychologists of the twentieth century, largely owing to his well-known hierarchy of needs. This highly influential theory was first proposed in his 1943 paper "A Theory of Human Motivation." Maslow suggested that the true driving force that motivates people in their search and evolution is the wish to satisfy certain needs and the deficiency they experience when they are unsated. As soon as one need is fulfilled, they seek to fulfill the next one. This search drives them to evolve from their more basic needs to the "higher needs" of psychic and spiritual growth.[14]

Maslow's earliest and most widespread version included five motivational needs, commonly presented as hierarchical levels within a pyramid. At the base of the pyramid, the individual is motivated to meet his or her physiological needs, such as air, food, water, shelter, warmth, and sleep. Next is safety, which includes security, stability, and freedom from fear. Above that group of needs, we experience our need for belonging and love, which is often satisfied by the company of friends, family, lovers, or coworkers. The last basic need is self-esteem, expressed as our search for achievement, mastery, independence, recognition, and respect. When any of these needs remain unmet for too long, Maslow claimed, the need to fulfill them will become stronger and more painful.

Maslow's original pyramid was topped by a "growth need," which he called self-actualization. This was the individual's need for the continual realization of all that one senses as a potential within oneself. Self-actualization could only be reached if all the

---

14   McLeod, "Hierarchy of Needs."

lower needs had been reasonably satisfied. Every person follows this natural evolution unless his or her progress has been disrupted by failure to meet lower-level needs. For example, if you divorced or lost your job, you might have found yourself fluctuating between levels of the pyramid.

Put simply, Maslow believed that if you had a full stomach, lived in a secure environment, felt that you belonged and were sufficiently respected by others, you would soon experience non-physiological hunger for realizing your personal potential, self-fulfillment, personal growth, and peak experiences.

During the 1970s, Maslow gradually expanded his five-level model into a seven-stage model and even an eight-stage one. First, he included cognitive and aesthetic needs: the need for knowledge and meaning and the need for appreciation of the world's beauty and the beauty expressed by the various arts. Later he added transcendental needs. In transcendence, the pinnacle of human development, he meant going beyond self-serving concerns and including humanity, other species, nature, and the cosmos within one's consciousness. It is our need for perspective and meaning beyond the personal that can fill us with the profound positivity of a broader awareness.[15] Maslow's last thought on human needs was that self-actualized persons will find themselves, in their search for wholeness, experiencing this highest, most refined need for a mystical vision and the attainment of an all-inclusive and compassionate universal consciousness.[16]

Although Maslow's hierarchy of needs has been well received as an important contribution to our understanding of human fulfillment, it has also raised some sound criticism. For instance, is

---

15   Ackerman, "What Is Self-Transcendence?"
16   Kowalski, "What Is Transcendence?"

it true that the lower needs must be satisfied *before* a person can actualize himself or herself?[17]

There are plenty of historical and cultural examples that tell us that this is not always the case. There are large numbers of people in India who live in extreme poverty and environmental insecurity while fulfilling higher-order needs, such as love, belongingness, and self-transcendence. Some artists, like Rembrandt and van Gogh, lived in poverty throughout their lifetime yet clearly achieved self-actualization. And the humanistic psychologist Viktor Frankl was able to find meaning and purpose in life while being tortured in a Nazi death camp.

Human needs do not always appear in an orderly fashion, one after another, since we are multilayered beings who possess different centers of perception and experience, all of which operate simultaneously and require our attention.

The Pyramid of Needs, According to the Seven Chakras

Maslow's hierarchy of needs inspired me to create a chakra-based pyramid of needs. Interestingly, when I set the eight-stage model that Maslow eventually built and the chakra model of needs side-by-side, they do not seem to be that different:

- Physiological and safety needs are the *root chakra* needs.
- Aesthetic needs are the *sacral chakra* needs.
- Esteem needs are the *solar plexus chakra* needs.
- Social needs are the *heart chakra* needs.
- Self-actualization needs are the *throat chakra* needs.

---

17   McLeod, "Hierarchy of Needs."

- Cognitive needs are the *third eye chakra* needs.
- Transcendence needs are the *crown chakra* needs.

If you think about it, it seems that Maslow's model intuitively captured the chakra journey of human fulfillment! The chakra knowledge tells us that all these physical, emotional, mental, and spiritual needs stem from these seven centers or layers of being. In fact, even Maslow's assumption that these needs evolve through an ever-refining ladder of development is congruent with the traditional view of chakras. According to the old concept of chakras, you climb these seven centers as if they were bars of a ladder; this means that as you learn the lesson of each, you leave it behind while keeping your eyes on the prize—the desired crown chakra, your ultimate goal.

But as soon as you begin to perceive chakras as different parts of your being that require continuous and simultaneous nourishment and activation, you no longer consider needs in this way. The pyramid of needs presented here departs from both Maslow's hierarchy and the traditional chakra ladder in that it is based on a philosophy of life that embraces all your needs at the same time. None of your needs are a luxury, and none of them can wait for a hypothetical future in which you have fully managed to meet other, more pressing needs.

If you want to be balanced and content, here is your map for tracking your sources of happiness and unhappiness. There is no need to guess. When you feel unhappy or unbalanced, simply take a look at this model and examine which needs you have neglected. All of these needs, both the material and the more refined ones, are essential for your complete being, from your most human elements all the way to the sublime spiritual being that you are.

It may be confusing at times to embrace all of your needs at the same time. People often find contradictory voices and desires inside themselves, each part pulling in a different direction. Fortunately, the seven-day chakra path ensures that you take care of all these needs in a way that consistently and increasingly balances the chakras and fills you with a growing sense of inner wholeness. By satiating your needs before they begin to ache, they will no longer need to pull in different directions to be heard—they will "know" that you are there, on the other side of the line, fully listening. Even your willingness to listen is enough to set in motion this process of inner balancing.

Your Needs, from Root to Crown

Here is your spectrum of needs according to the seven-day chakra path. As soon as you begin to follow the seven-day chakra path, you are free from the need to stick to this model since you'll be living it! However, studying this model can greatly inspire you, giving you another good reason to make this seven-day cycle a way of life. After all, you could think of each day as your opportunity to fulfill a certain set of needs. You can even declare every morning, "Today I'll be fulfilling my need for ..."

As you read through the following descriptions, I encourage you to evaluate how well you are currently meeting these needs in your life, from 1 to 100 percent. For a revealing experience, return to this section in a few weeks and reevaluate your percentages for evidence of your growth.

Root Chakra Needs: Physical Stability

Similarly to the first two foundational layers of Maslow's hierarchy, the chakra model opens with the root chakra's physiological and safety needs.

The first chakra conveys the genuine human need to feel stable ground under your feet. You may try to disregard this need, believing that you have transcended this stage by moving to higher realms of your being, but this is not a passing stage—it is an essential requirement for inner and outer security, your ability to trust the solidity of life's structures.

The first component of physical stability is being able to rely on your body. It is possible to walk on life's path with a fragile, burdened, or even diseased body—and sometimes, unfortunately, it is unavoidable. This would not necessarily prevent you from cultivating a rich intellectual life or profound spirituality, but feeling uncomfortable in your own body makes it so much harder. As much as possible, you need the body on your side: well-nourished, well-rested, flexible, and resilient.

The second component is the feeling that you have a home to return to and at least one framework to which you belong. This includes a roof over your head, but more broadly, some group affiliation and identification. If possible, maintaining family stability can greatly nurture the root chakra.

The third component of physical stability is the ability to rely on your life's structure and lifestyle: feeling that, in general, you are held by a healthy routine in a relatively quiet, calm, and supportive environment. Maintaining proper time management, which ensures that you take care of all your needs, is part of creating such an environment for yourself. Having a trusted income is an important ingredient as well.

Monday, the Day of Grounding, is devoted to the fulfillment of these root chakra needs.

Sacral Chakra Needs: Enjoyment

The second chakra needs to be nourished by life's juices. Life should be an enjoyable experience too, and there is nothing holy in suppressing this layer of yourself.

Your body is not merely a functional machine; it needs to feel alive, vibrant, and happy. A healthy sexuality is important, though it can easily take the form of physical intimacy and warmth. "Healthy" means a sensual sharing that is happy and loving rather than desirous or obsessive, which may leave the sacral chakra thirsty and dissatisfied.

Make sure that every week is dotted with touches of beauty, such as encounters with the arts or nature, as well as deep pleasure and joyous physical movement. As human beings, we are not meant to endure endless and uninterrupted routine, so peak experiences—intense, thrilling, playful, and adventurous—should "disrupt" your root chakra schedule every now and then. Even having free, purposeless breathing space and time is a form of healthy disruption of your routine.

Lastly, life without the joy of creativity—activating your imagination and spirit of inventiveness with passion and excitement— easily depletes your second chakra. This doesn't have to be a complex and purposeful project; even painting or writing a poem just for fun will do.

Tuesday, the Day of Joy, is devoted to the fulfillment of these sacral chakra needs.

Solar Plexus Chakra Needs: Power and Confidence

Many are embarrassed to acknowledge the fact that they need to feel powerful. However, this embarrassment leads to nothing but painful suppression. The third chakra tells us that we need to feel inwardly strong, confident, and resilient so that we can withstand all pressures, challenges, and power-tensions in social interactions and personal relationships.

Another empowering component is the feeling of having clearly defined goals and destinations. It is essential to know that you are confidently heading toward self-created futures with all your gathered energies and intentions. Succeeding in achieving at least some of your goals is crucial as well.

Although you are surely not meant or able to control all events and situations in life, you do need to feel "on top" of your life, capable of directing it through will and determination. Being unable to creatively influence the events in your life is a state of third chakra deprivation.

Wednesday, the Day of Power, is devoted to the fulfillment of these solar plexus chakra needs.

Heart Chakra Needs: Emotional Belonging

Our hearts need to engage in a mutual flow of intimate communication with others. You must not regard the longings you experience for external loving feedback as expressions of unhealthy dependency. The experience of deep emotional exchange—not necessarily a romantic one!—is an essential type of nourishment, especially when it includes not only receiving but also your own active giving. We all require the presence of some trusted others in our life, those who make us feel like we emotionally belong and who we can be positively attached to. A sufficient level of harmony in your personal relationships is also imperative, otherwise your home will fail to provide you with a much-needed emotional anchor.

A human heart needs to feel that it has some role and meaning in its contribution to the world. This is what Viktor Frankl recognized in his meaning-based psychology: to achieve psychological wholeness, you need to identify and define your existential meaning.[18]

Moreover, you need to feel that your efforts are met with appreciation, so there must be some supportive and affirming environment to recognize that. You try as hard as you can, including when you fall or go astray, and you need others (and yourself) to recognize that your attempts mean something after all.

Thursday, the Day of Love, is devoted to the fulfillment of these heart chakra needs.

Throat Chakra Needs: Authentic Self-Expression

It is healthy to wish that your voice is heard and acknowledged and that your authentic self will become visible in the world. Speaking your inner world is an integral part of engaging in human society and culture. When you suffocate your expression and conceal what you genuinely feel or think, you suppress a vital flow of participation and mutual influence.

You need to give voice to all that you strongly believe in. This does not imply that everyone should agree with you and respond with applause—actually, the more you dare to express, the more you expose yourself to criticism and resistance. But having even a

---

18   See Frankl, *Man's Search for Meaning*.

few people who are ready to listen and to seriously consider your thoughts and feelings is psychologically crucial.

It is essential to express not only ideas and feelings, but also visions that can eventually turn into a tangible reality in the world. It is unhealthy to remain stuck in your inner world, as rich as it may be, and to leave all that hidden potential unrealized. As a part of coming out, you need to strive to give form to inner visions and dreams, whether it is an artistic expression, a business enterprise, or new ways of improving and fulfilling your life and the lives of others.

Friday, the Day of Expression, is devoted to the fulfillment of these throat chakra needs.

Third Eye Chakra Needs: Mental Clarity

To achieve mental lucidity and order, people require states of deep silence. Without silence, our minds develop an overactive and frantic thinking that may even lead to self-destructive modes. Meditation is not really a recommendation; it is a need of the human mind that (quietly) screams from the depths of the sixth chakra.

When your mind is foggy, chaotic, and doubt-stricken, both your body and mind become disoriented and susceptible to unconscious influences. For this reason, you must be able to trust your own capacities of observation and judgment. You need your sixth chakra as a master that can confidently direct your being. It is thus vital to make use of any method that can sustain and promote the sharpness of your mind—from nutrition and supplementation to mental practices.

One of the major sources of mental clarity is the inspiration of great minds. Studying them through books and lectures can encourage you to attain your own peaks of intelligence and intellectual confidence. More than that, studying great minds helps you satisfy your deep sixth chakra need for mental nourishment, which is received through higher forms of knowledge and wisdom.

Saturday, the Day of Wisdom, is devoted to the fulfillment of these third eye chakra needs.

Crown Chakra Needs: Spiritual Union

The last set of needs can be equated with Maslow's transcendence, which also appears at the top of his hierarchy: our subtlest, transpersonal need.

As human beings who embody both divinity and humanity, you will remain hungry at the soul level until you experience oneness with the greater existence. It is the most refined human need to feel this type of belonging, this time not to a social structure, as in the root chakra, but to the universe and even to God.

An inherent part of the human condition is the experience of limitation: being trapped in the small box of a belief system, conditioning and thought patterns, unchanging routine, and even the boundaries of the human body. You need to feel that you can sometimes break free from this box, spread your wings and soar in the open and vast spaces of freedom and limitlessness. You must know that you have this option of retiring from the world from time to time, and not only in the unconscious form of deep sleep. Otherwise, a growing suffocation can easily creep in, causing an unexplainable suffering and different symptoms of physical, emotional, and mental imbalance.

The last need of the seventh chakra is being able to connect with a part of you that is unshakable and indestructible. Only your eternal spirit can grant you this: the experience that despite all physical fragility and dependency, you are, in essence, a divinity expressing itself through a human form.

Sunday, the Day of Spirit, is devoted to the fulfillment of these crown chakra needs.

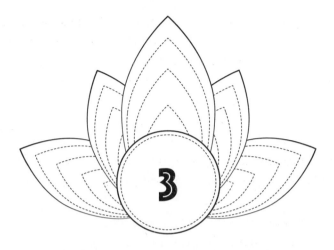

CHAKRA PERSONALITY TYPES AND THE SEVEN-DAY CYCLE

While practicing the seven-day chakra path, you will most likely discover that you are drawn toward certain days but reluctant to delve into others. In fact, I bet that while reading over the descriptions and recommended activities of each day, you will think, *This is what I'm doing!* or *This sounds like fun!* but also *A whole day only for that?* and *What a bore!* It is even likely that a certain day will seem intimidating and challenging to you.

Why is that?

One immediate answer is that the days you "like less" are not a part of your built-in personal structure. Another reasonable explanation is that your reluctance stems from personality imbalances that have formed lifestyle habits that are too stubborn to change.

And you can also put the blame on social, financial, and familial pressures that cause you to feel that technically, emotionally, and mentally, you cannot afford to "waste time" on such matters.

All of these answers—and perhaps others that have crossed your mind—are different pieces of the puzzle. But there is a bigger picture that contains all of them and much more. Interestingly, just as we have derived the key to a total and most fulfilling lifestyle from the seven-chakra system, we also find in it the key to explaining these personal biases: the seven chakra personality types.

The chakra personality type is an unusually individual aspect of the chakra system. The generally accepted use of the ancient chakra system is that all of us are meant to bring our seven energy centers to full balance and opening. This is not a false convention. Since each chakra represents an important dimension of your being, you can achieve lasting peace and completeness only when all seven dimensions are operative and synchronized. In many respects, the entire transformational and spiritual journey can be thought of as the process of balancing and awakening these seven centers of your being. That's exactly what the seven-day chakra path is all about!

Still, with all the balance in the world, even highly developed personalities experience and express different tastes and inclinations. You could imagine that someone like Mother Teresa would be particularly fond of Thursday, the Day of Love, and that someone like Albert Einstein would prefer to indulge in the mind-broadening delights of Saturday, the Day of Wisdom. The fact that we energize all our chakras does not mean that having some of them more active than others is a sign of weakness or imbalance. On the contrary: this may be an indication of a wonderful capacity of the chakras to reflect your deepest, most essential personality—what I regard as the "soul-print."

While we are all blessed with seven centers, each of us has a specific inborn and unchanging design which makes one chakra the leader of our entire character. Two more chakras—a secondary one and a supportive one—complete the picture by creating an interplay of three main forces that give shape to our personality.[19] This means that your personal bias toward some of the days as well as your wish to avoid others are not mistakes that need to be corrected; you will obviously feel most comfortable with the days that resemble your natural chakra design and have mixed feelings in relation to the days that do not resonate with this design.

Remember that chakras are manifestations of the seven dimensions of life. Each is like a gateway through which we connect with its corresponding dimension (root chakra/grounding, sacral chakra/joy, solar plexus chakra/power, and so on). But people are built in such a way that we are more effortlessly connected with three aspects of life and the universe. This fact is crucial: it determines your meaning in life, your unique form of happiness, and your expression and fulfillment in the world. We cannot and shouldn't demonstrate the entire spectrum of the seven dimensions; through your personal example, you are destined to manifest only a few of the seven dimensions, but in the most spectacular way possible.

This is perhaps the first message of the chakra personality types: there is not one prescription for happiness, but seven major ones. (And 252 more nuanced prescriptions for happiness

---

19   If you wish to investigate further, read my book *The Seven Chakra Personality Types.*

if you consider each three-chakra structure combination!) You may be fascinated with the latest bestselling book on happiness and self-fulfillment, yet it will not necessarily be *your* book. What makes *my* life meaningful may not trigger your own meaning-seeking impulse at all, and vice versa. This is because your most authentic inclinations and passions derive from the dimensions you are naturally most drawn to. Only when you faithfully follow them will you be able to get a hold of your own unique expression in life.

This is the intriguing paradox that we need to settle in this chapter: How is it possible to simultaneously respect your cosmos-given preferences *and* use this seven-day cycle as your ultimate form of self-fulfillment? Although at first this can seem like a startling riddle, the answers you will receive by the end of the chapter are likely to enhance and deepen your weekly experience even more.

A Brief Overview of the Individual Chakra Types

One easy way of identifying your three strongest chakras is by noting which of the chakra days you feel most comfortable with upon your first reading. This self-diagnosis can be complemented by reading the following overview of the seven personalities. If you are intrigued by the concept or if you feel that you require more elaborate descriptions to identify yourself, read my book *The Seven Chakra Personality Types.*

Root Chakra Personality Type: Builders

Builders are guided by the instinctual and biological center located in the root chakra. They embody the wisdom of the physical world and its harmonious structures. Like forever-busy ants, they build the world around them, creating order and aspiring to establish peace in their surroundings. They enjoy following laws, are proudly traditional, and feel naturally drawn to preserve the past and to honor their roots.

As fervent believers in structure, they like belonging to collectives and love family and community life. They lead a steady life, building brick-by-brick toward increasing stability and solidity. Since "God is in the details," they appreciate the significance of the smallest, most mundane details and technicalities. They are not interested in the "why" of things but more in the "how": how the world works and what can make it work even better.

Builders love routine and are able to do the same thing for a long time. They are diligent, accurate, serious, and reliable personalities. But they can also be rigid, over-structured, uninventive, slow, and lethargic. They don't like surprises or sudden changes and avoid risks. They can also be anxious, territorial, and possessive.

Their presence in the world gifts us with the wisdom of balance, structure, and grounding. They are most fulfilled by functioning as a part of a structure, serving a community, and spending time with family. They can benefit, however, from energizing activities and foods, avoiding resting too much, accepting and initiating changes, and some measure of humor and laughter.

Sacral Chakra Personality Type: Artists

Artists are guided by the impulsive center located in the sacral chakra. They embody this chakra of joy, feeling, and passion that is deeply connected to life's juices and colors. For them, life is a playground—a place for peak experiences and experimentation. Convinced that life must always be exciting, they hover over life's different experiences like butterflies. They are true lovers of life, filled with bubbling life force, but their energy is like a flare: intense and short-lived. Hence, they live only in the now, not paying much attention to long-term purposes and commitments.

For Artists, everything is either interesting or boring. They experience constant ups and downs, deep joys and profound depressions, living messily without clear direction. They possess an artistic and poetic soul, capable of identifying the full spectrum of feelings more than anyone else. They are drawn to beauty and their senses are wide awake. They learn about the world through their bodies and evaluate the truthfulness of knowledge and ideas according to their gut feelings. In interaction, they are talkative, humorous, and intimate, but also self-centered and unreliable. Like the fictional Peter Pan who wishes to remain a child and never age, Artists fear growing up and shirk commitments. As free-hearted individuals who detest structure and discipline, they insist on flowing freely throughout life. Deep down, they can sometimes be sad clowns.

Artists teach us how to feel and experience deeply and how to lead a life of passion. They are fulfilled through artistic and physical expression. Their balance is achieved by reducing disorder, moodiness, and destructive behavior and learning to love and commit.

Solar Plexus Chakra Personality Type: Achievers

Achievers are governed by the center of will located in the solar plexus chakra. They embody this fiery chakra that determines everyone's level of inner power, resolution, and strength of will. Exploding with well-targeted energy, they are highly competitive and uncompromising winners at heart. For them, life is a potential that is fulfilled by marking those mountaintops worthy of reaching. They live from one achievement to another and search for destinations that can make them stand out and excel. They are warriors who perceive life as a play of power and love trials of self-overcoming. They are always busy and enjoy having tight schedules; they sometimes consider nights an unwelcome interruption.

Achievers are endowed with great strategic intelligence. But often their overflowing energy keeps them attached to achieving for the sake of achieving while remaining inwardly dissatisfied and forever wanting more. Their focus on their goals can make them unemotional, controlling, aggressive, and arrogant. This may damage their relationships, as they disregard others' feelings as well.

This personality can inspire others to seek out and define their own goals and destinations—to unwaveringly move toward self-realization and victory, even if this requires overcoming self-limitations and inhibitions. Achievers are fulfilled by accepting their workaholic nature and setting and declaring clear destinations. However, they should direct their ambitions for the greater good and develop compassion toward others' needs. They should also be cautious not to lead an unbalanced lifestyle and burn their energies out; they can do this by agreeing to relax and disengage from action sometimes.

Heart Chakra Personality Type: Caretakers

Caretakers are governed by the emotional center located in the heart chakra. They embody this chakra of relationships that is centered on the emotional interaction between "me" and "the other" and the aspiration to make two into one. For Caretakers, love is the only fulfillment. They fervently seek to unite opposing sides and establish common ground. Their mind is naturally occupied with thoughts about their relationships. In quarrels, they are not troubled by who is right, but by the disharmony itself. They are soft, gentle, peace-loving, and relaxing characters who love cultivating heart-to-heart communication. They are also incurably optimistic and naive, believing that people are good by nature. They are also drawn to service and compassionate acts.

Caretakers are almost always fulfilled through a certain ultimate other to whom they are fully devoted. As such, they are emotionally dependent because they require the other's approval to have their existence validated. They have a profound need to be loved; they sometimes serve (and even sacrifice themselves) only to receive emotional recognition. They can be jealous, possessive, demanding, hypersensitive, and even self-centered. Usually, they don't possess sufficient drive or ambition of their own.

Caretakers demonstrate the importance of the heart center in human life and the need to cultivate intimacy, acceptance, compassion, and empathy. They are fulfilled by becoming healers or peacemakers, uniting people and bringing hope to their lives, and serving a higher purpose. They achieve balance by calming their stormy emotions, developing independence, and finding channels for love and closeness beyond their ultimate other.

Throat Chakra Personality Type: Speakers

Speakers are guided by the center of communication located in the throat chakra. They embody this chakra of expression that creates bridges between different worlds through words and other means of communication. For Speakers, the world is a place for influence, an opportunity for the effective expression of their inner truths and values. They passionately search for ways to change the world by disseminating inspiring ideas. They live in visions of far-off futures and dreams that are bigger than life. They are most fulfilled when they change someone's life and are comfortable standing in front of audiences. In interaction, they are less interested in intimacy and more in leading people to accept their own convictions and guidance. As good salespeople, they know how to identify the needs of others. They can be charismatic educators and teachers, representatives of systems, and creators of networks and organizations.

Speakers tend to possess unclear personalities: like chameleons, they adjust to any environment. They can be manipulative, righteous, uncaring, and controlling since everything has to happen according to their plan. Dreaming big can easily turn into dreaminess, focusing on the vision without taking the small and realistic steps toward its manifestation. They can also be lazy, encouraging others to do their own work.

Speakers inspire us to dare to dream—to insist on developing our greater visions and holding on to them. They are fulfilled by becoming teachers, affecting people's lives, and forming connections between different people and systems of thought. They can become balanced by learning to be less controlling and more flexible. They also need to pay attention to people's feelings and agree to be influenced by others.

Third Eye Chakra Personality Type: Thinkers

Thinkers are guided by the intellectual center located in the third-eye chakra. They embody this chakra of wisdom that enables us to see into the hidden reality of life's mysteries. For Thinkers, life is an exciting riddle seeking to be unraveled. Their greatest happiness is found in insight and understanding and so, naturally, books are their closest companions. They live inside their minds, and their experience of life is centered on the richness of their thought. They are observers and listeners of the human world, and even their own emotional experience is a subject of research. This makes them good scientists and philosophers, interested in the "why" of things. Thinkers look for some "theory of everything" that can settle life's greatest questions. They are brilliant, original, and profound. They are also strong individuals who avoid crowds and crowd mentality and can easily stay alone in one room without disturbance for days on end.

As bodiless observers of life, Thinkers are never really here. They are quite helpless in handling reality and do everything they can to avoid engaging too much. Thinking, for them, is like experiencing. They are also unemotional and asocial and can be highly critical and arrogant.

Thinkers reveal to us the ecstasy of deep thinking and the beauty and potential of having a reflective and inquisitive mind. They should not listen to those who tell them to get out of their head and start living—their fulfillment lies in the domains of pure research, away from people and mundane fuss. However, they should sometimes leave the house to immerse in nature, physical activity, social interaction, and experiences without thinking.

Crown Chakra Personality Type: Yogis

Yogis are governed by the spiritual center located in the crown chakra. They embody this chakra of transcendence that connects humans with the infinite, beyond the ephemeral world of form. For Yogis, life is nothing but a play of spirit. Their role in it is to become free from earthly bondage and to return to their true home. This rare personality is purely interested in the inner journey, passionately drawn to the hidden realms of consciousness and to the energetic and astral planes. They consider mundane life a distraction and a test for the soul that yearns for liberation. This makes their meditation natural and effortless. Yogis often find themselves as priests, monks, and renunciates. When they lead a conventional lifestyle, they make their home their cave. They are harmless and gentle and possess a transparent personality. They are also not possessive, naturally unattached, and devoid of clear wills and urges. They are simpleminded and singleminded, and they feel relaxed in existing traditions.

This transparency, however, makes Yogis vulnerable and hypersensitive. Since they perceive the demands of human life as a nuisance, they attempt to avoid all conflict and challenge and find it hard to commit to work and relationships. They hope that others can do the work for them, and this often ends in poverty and dependency. In a way, they are confused and disoriented when they are not in ashrams and monasteries.

Yogis encourage us to sometimes step aside from the rat race, enter meditation and silence, and contact life's unchanging essence. They are fulfilled by following their inner calling to focus on the divine and the inner journey. They should, however, balance themselves by appreciating the spiritual value of life, remaining grounded, and accepting certain responsibilities.

· · · · ·

Perhaps you have identified yourself in one, two, or even three of these descriptions. This usually feels like an inner smile of self-recognition that spreads within your being. Remember that none of us is 100 percent one type—your core personality is a blend of three chakras in varying degrees of intensity. By comparing these instances of self-identification with the days that make you feel at home, you will most likely reach your unique three-type structure.

The following questionnaire will help you identify your chakra type.

Identifying Your Chakra Personality Type: A Questionnaire

This questionnaire contains twenty-five questions. For each question there are seven possible answers. You are invited to select one or two relevant answers to each question.

The numbers that have been repeated the most comprise your winning chakra, second winner, and third winner. For instance, if you selected answer c. fifteen times, answer a. ten times, and answer d. nine times, you are likely the solar plexus chakra personality type, the Achiever, with a secondary type of the Builder, and a supportive type of a Caretaker.

Although this may not be the complete picture of your chakra type constitution—sometimes this process requires some more rigorous soul-searching—the results will surely propel you in the right direction.

1. Select the statement you identify with the most.

    a. The world is an opportunity for building something solid—diligently and patiently establishing stability, ground, and peace of mind.

    b. The world is a field of endless possible adventures and excitements and we are here to fully experience all of them, hopefully missing nothing.

c. The world is an opportunity for bringing the best out of myself, becoming a success story, and coming out victorious.

d. The world is a space of emotional bonding, and we are here to realize our maximum potential as love in a human form.

e. The world is an opportunity to bring out your message, express your truest voice, and influence others' lives.

f. The world is a space of endless learning and knowledge and our role in it is to stretch our intelligence and understanding as much as possible.

g. The world is an opportunity for a profound inner journey of spiritual liberation and transcendence.

2. What would you say is the most active part of you?

a. The earthly, grounded, and instinctual part of my being.

b. My feelings, impulses, and the intelligence of my body.

c. My willpower and ambition.

d. My deep emotional world.

e. My voice, expression, and communication.

f. My mind and intellect.

g. The spiritual part of my being.

3. Which image immediately makes you feel like you are in the right place?

a. A beautiful house, a garden, and prosperous land.

b. Someone dancing in a trancelike, ecstatic state at a nature party.

c. Climbing a mountaintop, nearly reaching the peak.

d. Two people's hands entwining and caressing each other.

e. A speaker in a big lecture hall facing a large crowd.

f. A library and a lone writer sitting in it, immersed in their own world.

g. A monk in deep meditation.

4. My ideal way of sharing my being with others is …

a. Serving the needs of my family and community with my skills and abilities.

b. Having fun, sharing ecstasy, dancing, and experiencing physical and sensual joy.

c. Striving together toward some shared target with effort and determination.

d. A one-on-one personal and intimate sharing in which we open our hearts to one another.

e. Guiding others or discussing and creating a grand vision with them.

f. Engaging in a profound philosophical discussion with a thoughtful person.

g. Meditating, praying, and just being with others who are spiritually oriented.

5. The best way I could spend my time is by …

a. Making small actions and plans that put life into order and balance.

b. Spending time outdoors, moving and breathing the moment deep into my being.

c. Making sure that everything I do can lead me to my goal.

d. Helping someone and making sure they are happy.

e. Writing or recording a message that could change people's lives.

f. Delving into a book by a great philosopher.

g. Watching a video of a spiritual or religious teacher.

6. Since childhood, my main connection with the world has been through …

a. My search for belonging and my role in the systems of the world.

b. Playfulness and experimentation.

c. Winning in different competitions and platforms.

d. Strong feelings toward certain others.

e. Educating and leading others.

f. Distant observation and quiet, inner study.

g. Indifference and unbelonging.

7. Others would say that I am …

a. Diligent, serious, responsible, cautious, and accurate.

b. Jumpy, intense, passionate, humorous, and always hunting for a new experience.

c. Ambitious, driven, focused, busy, and competitive.

d. Emotional, sensitive, caring, helpful, and kindhearted.

e. Inquisitive, controlling, intense, idealistic, and expressive.

f. Wise, silent, remote, deep, and wakeful.

g. Spiritual, introverted, unearthly, gentle, and spacey.

8. At heart, I am a …

    a. Hard worker.

    b. Dancer.

    c. Warrior.

    d. Lover.

    e. Communicator.

    f. Philosopher.

    g. Meditator.

9. I am …

    a. Slow and careful.

    b. Quick and careless.

    c. Persistent and pushy.

    d. Mild and harmonious.

    e. Intense and engaging.

    f. Distant and observant.

    g. Dreamy and spacey.

10. Choose the word that you respond the most to.

    a. Foundation.

    b. Passion.

    c. Victory.

    d. Love.

    e. Vision.

    f. Wisdom.

    g. Silence.

11. Which building sounds the most interesting and impressive to you?

    a. An ancient history museum.

    b. A Gaudi building.

    c. A skyscraper.

    d. A home for the poor.

    e. A congress hall.

    f. A university.

    g. An ashram or a monastery.

12. When I leave this world, I want to know that…

    a. I have benefited and contributed to my family, community, and people.

    b. I have experienced life totally and let it in fully.

    c. I have achieved the highest goals I set for myself.

    d. I have loved strongly enough.

    e. I have left behind a legacy of influence and impact.

    f. I have understood some of life's hidden mysteries.

    g. I have experienced my innermost spirit.

13. Which of these negative attributes characterizes you the most?

   a. Overcautious.

   b. Uncommitted.

   c. Angry.

   d. Needy.

   e. Controlling.

   f. Arrogant.

   g. Detached.

14. How do you feel when you read the following statement? "I love dealing with details—calculations and figures, materials and accurate planning, pieces of information, and schedules."

   a. Yes!

   b. No, dealing with details makes me want to fly away. I love doing nothing!

   c. Yes, but only if this leads me to some clear and powerful goal.

   d. Yes, but only if it clearly helps me serve someone I love.

   e. No, I would rather leap to the vision at the edge of my imagination.

   f. No, small details have no intelligence or depth in them.

   g. No, earthly life has no spiritual meaning.

15. When an overwhelming negative emotion arises in me, I…

    a. Do anything I can to calm it down and put myself back together.

    b. Become one with it, totally experience it, and quickly return to joy.

    c. Take it out on my surroundings.

    d. Become overwhelmed, and I struggle to transform it into harmony.

    e. Try to control and suffocate it.

    f. Investigate it as a scientist.

    g. Meditate.

16. How much do you like change and mobility in life (as opposed to routine and permanence)?

    a. Strong changes feel unhealthy and destabilizing for me. I prefer slow and gradual building.

    b. Change is my middle name. I always feel on fire and can't stand routine!

    c. I don't like disruptions, but I know how to adjust them to my plans.

    d. I am fine with changes as long as I get to keep all my loved ones with me.

    e. I get confused when things change and collide with the dream inside me.

    f. I prefer to create a routine that allows me to freely delve into my mental life.

    g. I don't initiate changes, but I can accept changes when they come as God's will.

17. How would you describe your type and level of energy?

    a. Slow and persistent, like low fire.

    b. Rapid, quick, and physical, like a flare.

    c. Massive and uncompromising, like a bulldozer.

    d. Gentle and soft, like a breeze.

    e. Intense and wakeful.

    f. Mainly concentrated in my head, not so physical.

    g. Airy, like levitation.

18. I feel most alive when…

    a. I manage to grasp the inner mechanism of something.

    b. I am in a creative expression.

    c. I manage to remove obstacles and make a step forward.

    d. I am in a state of intimacy and bonding.

    e. I manage to influence and affect the lives of others.

    f. I have new and brilliant insights.

    g. I manage to enter deep states of consciousness.

19. How do you feel when you read the following statement? "I want to change the world!"

    a. My aspirations are not that great. I want to know that I benefit others and society at large.

    b. Far from it. I just want to be myself and express creatively and authentically.

    c. I want to conquer the world!

    d. I just spread love with all my heart. Whatever happens, happens.

e. Yes; by spreading my ideas, visions, and creations, I dream of creating a global impact.

f. My thoughts and ideas are far too deep to change the common people.

g. World change is none of my concern. I am only occupied with the eternal.

20. Think for a moment of the color that best represents your deepest, innermost being (as opposed to your "favorite" color).

a. Deep red.

b. Fizzy orange.

c. Radiant yellow.

d. Soft and light green.

e. Deep and intense blue.

f. Deep and mysterious purple.

g. Bright white; colorless.

21. Choose your most cherished values.

a. Respect, loyalty, patience.

b. Joy, totality, beauty.

c. Courage, perseverance, dignity.

d. Compassion, friendship, harmony.

e. Authenticity, autonomy, self-expression.

f. Intelligence, clarity, depth.

g. Purity, nonattachment, freedom.

22. How do you feel when you read the following statement? "I love being a part of a larger unit like a tradition, family, community, or nation. It feels healthy and supportive."

    a. Perfectly accurate.

    b. Not at all! I avoid frameworks that limit my freedom of choice and experience.

    c. I appreciate structures, but it is most important for me to stand out and be myself.

    d. Structures are wonderful as long as they are opportunities for love.

    e. I am more interested in my dreams about better, even utopian, communities.

    f. Such structures are for common people. I prefer to research this phenomenon.

    g. Only if these larger units are spiritual and support spirituality.

23. How much do you like long-term projects and lifetime commitments?

    a. A lot—as long as they are relaxed and secure processes.

    b. The very idea terrifies me. I feel like I'm in a cage.

    c. I like them as long as they lead to some successful end and are constantly growing and expanding.

    d. I like them, but they need to be essentially emotional commitments.

    e. I like them, but only if they include a vision that thrills me and never stifles my dreams.

f. I like them if they are intellectual by nature and lead to ever-growing depths.

g. My only lifelong commitment is to my spiritual journey.

24. Choose the figure that you relate to the most.

a. Thomas Alva Edison, inventor.

b. Jim Morrison, rock legend and poet.

c. Ernesto "Che" Guevara, warrior and revolutionary.

d. Mother Teresa, missionary of charity.

e. Martin Luther King Jr., speaker and leader.

f. Sigmund Freud, psychologist and theorist.

g. Francis of Assisi, saint.

25. Which historical revolution impresses you the most?

a. The agricultural or industrial revolution.

b. The social revolution of the '60s (flower children).

c. The second World War victory.

d. Nonviolent peace movements like Gandhi's and King's.

e. The emergence of democracy in ancient Athens.

f. Ancient Greek philosophy.

g. The emergence of teachers like the Buddha or Jesus.

Accept Yourself, but Also Balance Yourself

The benefits of recognizing your type are great. The most obvious benefit is a deeper understanding of your strengths and limitations, virtues and struggles. We tend to over-personalize our personality structures, but the chakra system tells us that our foundational personalities belong to more general patterns, almost like the different forces of nature.

As a direct result of this self-understanding, a gateway opens, leading us to a truly liberating self-acceptance. Your type is not really different from being a zebra or an elephant. Has the thought that there is something wrong with zebras ever crossed your mind? Have you ever complained about the zebra's stripes or tail, thinking that it should transform itself into an elephant? In the case of zebras, this thought sounds ridiculous, but when it comes to our own personality patterns, many feel that there are better patterns and hope that one day they will become an elephant.

The chakra types make it possible for us to finally relax into our natural programming and even to perceive our so-called shortcomings in a more understanding light, realizing that every natural pattern must have limitations. Take a step further and you will see how this self-acceptance can extend to include the natural design of others around us. Through the lens of this system, you are able to observe people with compassionate eyes. Knowing that they experience life differently as a result of a natural program, you no longer expect them to be like you and to share your values and choices. You can even enjoy their otherness, since it is packed with gifts and wisdom that balance and inspire your being.

The main instruction of the seven chakra personality types is that we should all relax into our unique pattern and follow its innate inclinations and passions. These inclinations and passions are deeply connected with the possibility of realizing our unique type of happiness and meaning in life. And yet, having embraced the precious gifts of self-acceptance and self-fulfillment, we should acknowledge that our constitution suffers from certain imbalances and unhealthy excesses. Actually, each chakra type tends to have an overflow of its characteristics. So, attaching ourselves to our natural design without restraint can damage and sometimes even endanger us. More than that, it can limit and inhibit the full expression of our unique personality type.

At this point, the seven-day cycle enters the picture.

Those days that feel to you like going against the stream of your effortless inclinations and habits are exactly your weekly opportunities to balance your excesses and empower your self-expression. Of course, our brain's first reaction to coming out of its comfort zone is resistance. A solar plexus chakra type—an Achiever—will most vehemently resist Tuesdays, which are wholly dedicated to purposeless joy; Thursdays, which are devoted to matters of the heart and intimate communion; and Sundays, which are a pure immersion in the spirit. A heart chakra type—a Caretaker—will be reluctant to dip his or her toes in the water of Wednesdays, which call for defining and pursuing goals and the cultivation of self-independence, or Saturdays, which prefer intellectual expansion to the sweetness of emotions. And think of the poor Yogi—a crown chakra type—who needs to engage in strengthening earthly foundations on Monday or in self-expression and manifestation on Fridays! In general, the more airy types—the Artists, Caretakers, Thinkers, and Yogis—dislike the active and earthly aspects of the seven-day cycle, whereas natural-born doers—the Builders, Achievers, and Speakers—wrinkle their noses when they think of the more reflective, emotional, and experiential days.

While these immediate resistances are understandable, consider for a moment an Achiever who unstoppably works day and night, renouncing purposeless joy, heart communion, and immersion in spirit. Sooner or later, this will lead to a severe burnout, or perhaps to feelings of frustration and a growing doubt that this endless marathon that has no finish line is worth the trouble. Such an Achiever will become much angrier. They will be more inclined to develop addictions and use relieving substances, like alcohol, drugs, and junk food, which will make them more alienated from their peers, family, and friends. The great irony is that avoiding areas of balance and empowerment will eventually prevent the Achiever from finding meaning and happiness in the solar plexus chakra endeavor. As a matter of fact, avoiding these areas can keep the Achiever from achieving at all.

Using the Seven-Day Cycle to Empower Your Type

The seven-day chakra path integrates the whole-human awakening of the seven chakras with the individual fulfillment of your chakra type. On the one hand, each week is a total journey that embraces all seven aspects of your being. On the other hand, the fact that you have "stronger" days and "weaker" days is also taken into consideration—not as an obstacle that needs to be removed, but as a meaningful reality that provides you with one more reason to make this cycle your new routine.

The weak days of your week are not enemies that interfere with your life mission. These days that you like less may be days that broaden your horizons and provoke further growth (if you are a Builder). Or days that empower your more active and involved aspects (if you are an Artist or a Caretaker). Or days that cool you down (if you are a fiery Achiever). Or days that ground your being in the actuality of human experience (if you are a dreamy Speaker, Thinker, or Yogi).

When you consider the relevance of these days to your unique personality and perceive them as a necessary part of your individual process of balance and empowerment, you start engaging in them wholeheartedly. On your stronger days you celebrate your natural design, and on your more challenging days you correct its excesses, keep it healthy, and round it out. No doubt, those around you will also be grateful to have you as a more complete "you."

To initiate your conscious work with this reality of natural and unnatural days, create a list of your strong days—hopefully, the list will consist of at least three! Then, take a look at this list. It is easy to guess that at this point in time, these strong days are really what you are occupied with—physically, emotionally, and mentally—throughout most of your regular seven-day cycle. Since you are effortlessly inclined toward pursuing the passions of these days, they form many of your habits and determine the flow of your week. Try to explain, ideally in a written form, why these days are your strongest and most obvious preference.

It is, however, important to bear in mind that even these days should not be taken for granted as elements that you have already fully mastered. It is possible that you are currently fulfilling only around 20 or 30 percent of their dormant potential! Both your understanding and experience of your stronger days can be deepened. So, in this writing practice, contemplate the ways each of these days could become a further revelation beyond your familiar boundaries and habits.

Now move on to the second half of your practice and create a list of your more challenging and neglected days. Take the time to contemplate each of them separately—and, if you find a common thread, use it to deepen your insight into the meaning of these days. Patiently, answer the following questions about each of the days:

- Why do I feel that this day is unnatural? Is there also some fear involved in my reluctance?

- How could I use this day to balance, heal, cool down, or empower my being?

- What can this day show me or teach me?

- What forces and qualities can this day awaken in me?

- In what way can this day be a missing piece in the puzzle of my being?

Your work is done when you feel that you genuinely appreciate and love these days. It is all about developing an *emotional connection* with them. You can imagine the strong days as the core of your being while the "weak" days surround this core as supporters. Feel how this constellation forms a complete picture of your being in its most balanced and rounded form. You can even create a drawing that makes this vision more tangible.

Equipped with the knowledge of the chakra personality types, you now know that your built-in inclinations are precious discoveries of your soul design. But they shine even more when held by a week that is truly holistic.

Chakra Meditations

Now that you have explored the individual dimension of your own chakra system, it is time to learn two methods that instantly enkindle the chakra system as a whole. These will prepare you for your dive into your new way of holistic life.

Smiling into Your Chakras Meditation

This self-guided meditation is one of the easiest, most effective ways to stimulate the individual chakras as well as the chakra system as a whole. It releases the healing and soothing power of these seven energy centers assisted by one of the greatest healers in the world: your smile.

By now, there is sufficient scientific evidence that smiling, even deliberately, activates neural messaging that benefits health and happiness: it activates the release of neuropeptides that work toward fighting off stress as well as the "feel-good" neurotransmitters—dopamine, endorphins, and serotonin.[20] This relaxes your body, lowers your heart rate and blood pressure, lengthens your lifespan, and—thanks to the endorphins—even acts as a natural pain reliever. There is absolutely no need to wait for a situation that would trigger a smile; the very effect is achieved by the decision to smile. As Buddhist teacher Thich Nhat Hanh puts it, "Sometimes your joy is the source of your smile, but sometimes your smile can be the source of your joy." Of particular relevance is one study published in the journal *Neuropsychologia*, which reported that seeing a smiling face activates our orbitofrontal cortex, the region of the brain that processes sensory rewards. That means we feel rewarded when smiled at.[21]

In this meditation we invoke a smiling and rewarding face, respond to it, and—using its essence—turn it into an inner smile that can vitalize the chakras. This meditation, loosely based on the Taoist meditation called "the inner smile meditation" and popularized by Taoist master Mantak Chia, is adapted here to the world of chakras.

---

20   Riggio, "Magic in Your Smile."
21   Riggio, "Magic in Your Smile."

There are two ways to apply this meditation to the seven-day chakra path: as activation of all seven chakras or as a one-chakra activation. As a complete process that activates all seven chakras, it suits Monday, the Day of Grounding, or Sunday, the Day of Spirit. Monday is a good day to structure your life, so the seven-chakra activation can help by strengthening your energetic and physical foundations. Sunday is the day when you move beyond all chakras to rest in the completeness of your being, and that is why full-chakra activation supports this experience of inner completeness. For a one-chakra activation, simply focus on an individual chakra, taking time to fully steep your chosen chakra in the smiling energy.

Carefully read the meditation's instructions and then close your eyes and guide yourself through this chakra journey. You can also record yourself reading the meditation and follow along, or you can follow my guided meditation of "Smiling into Your Chakras" on YouTube.[22]

• • • • •

As you breathe slowly and deeply, letting your body relax more and more with every breath you take, place your attention on the area of the lower forehead where the sixth chakra, the third eye, is located. In front of the sixth chakra, visualize a vivid image that best represents to you the deepest or happiest smile you can imagine. This could be the smile of a child (perhaps your child); your own smile at a certain point in time, in which you were the happiest or most content; the smile of an admired figure; the known Mona

---

22   https://www.youtube.com/watch?v=h3YKwLgv_sw.

Lisa subtle smile; or the smile of the Buddha as depicted in some of his statues.

Picturing the smile as vividly as possible, feel this joy and inner knowing that you find irresistible. You might feel tempted to smile yourself, at least inwardly.

Now bring this image to maximum clarity, then drop the image and remain only with the essence or the energy of this smile. Feel how the essence of this smile begins to pour into your lower forehead, as if your sixth chakra has become a funnel that enables this energy to flow into your head.

Drawing on this smiling energy, smile into the area of the top of your head, as if you are injecting this smile that now spreads and makes the area itself smile. Include the two hemispheres of the brain and the space between them. Even if you are bewildered by the image of a smiling brain, realize how that image relaxes the brain and the entire upper skull.

Allow more of the smiling energy to flow through the third eye and use it to smile into your lower forehead. As a result, feel how the forehead eases into a smile from its center, relaxing any mental tension that may have accumulated.

Keep on letting this smiling energy pour in until it drips from the lower forehead into the area at the base of the throat. Use it to smile into the throat so that it is filled with this energy. Feel how an inner smile begins to spread, relieving any tension in the related areas of the neck and jaw.

Let the smiling energy flow downward, like a gentle stream, all the way to the lower center of your chest. Smile into your heart and visualize how, in response, an inner smile spreads there also, from the center of your chest throughout your entire torso and even the shoulders. It is important to have your heart smile. Feel how this soothes any heartache and how your chest widens and breathes more fully and deeply, opening up to feelings, people, and life.

Now let the smiling energy flow to the area of the solar plexus, where the third chakra is located. Smile into your solar plexus and feel how this compelling inner smile stretches and gently fills the entire upper belly. Allow the smiling belly to relieve any stored pressure in the solar plexus as well as the digestive system. Yes, even bellies can smile!

As the smiling energy keeps on streaming down, it reaches the area of the pubic bone, just above the genitals, where the sacral chakra is located. Feel how you are internalizing the energy of the inner smile to smile into your pelvis. Let it sweeten and open up the entire pelvic region with a smile that begins in the center of the lower abdomen and stretches in all directions.

Finally, the smiling energy descends to the area of the perineum, between the genitals and the anus, where the root chakra is located. Smile into the perineum and let a soft smile unfold there, spreading all the way to the legs, thighs, knees, and feet, transforming every bit of tension.

Swiftly smile into your chakras, one after another, this time in the upward direction. Once again, smile into the perineum, lower abdomen, solar plexus, center of the chest, base of the throat, lower forehead, and upper scalp. Feel how you enkindle each and every center through these brief smiles.

With your seven chakras grinning, visualize how they unify and become one big inner smile that covers the entire body from head to toe. Allow the remaining smiling energy to be absorbed in your body until you yourself become this unbeatable smile.

Smile at yourself, others, and the entire world, softly greeting everything and everyone. Let this inner smile settle in your mouth, *cheeks, and eyes, bringing you to a physical, authentic smile. This is unlike the social smile of politeness or the smile that spreads on your face when you are triggered by something that pleases you. Rather, it is a smile that emerges from the richness of your awakened being and overflowing chakras, so nothing can take it away from you.*

Slowly and gently open your eyes, keeping the smiling presence in you as an active ingredient for the remainder of your day.

Chakra Flowering Meditation

Balanced chakras resemble open flowers: blooming from the central column that pierces through the center of our body, they unfold at the frontal part of our body, uninhibitedly facing and welcoming the world. The following self-guided meditation imitates this subtle mechanism of the balanced state of the chakras. Similar to the power of a deliberate smile, imitating a balanced state temporarily causes it to come into being.

A chakra feels healthy, aligned, and flowing when its energy readily opens up to the world, exposing its inner beauty; when it is willing to be nurtured by life's light and air and to be fully exposed, even in the face of challenges and pain.

On the other hand, a chakra turns sick, hollow, malnourished, and blocked when its energy is withdrawn. Unbalanced chakras have their energy collapse into the central column, like a closed flower. They literally turn their back on the world, refusing to be visible and to allow full participation in life.

Chakra flowering is a gentle meditation that encourages the chakras to come out of their hiding place within the central channel and bloom at their kshetram. It is as effective as the previous meditation in quickly stimulating the chakra system. Similarly, you can use this meditation on a daily basis to activate an individual chakra or on either Monday or Sunday as a way to promote wholeness in the body-mind system.

Carefully read the meditation's instructions and then close your eyes and guide yourself through this chakra journey. You can also record yourself reading the meditation and follow along, or you can follow my guided meditation of "Chakra Flowering Meditation" on YouTube.[23]

• • • • •

As you breathe slowly and deeply, letting your body relax more and more with every breath you take, connect with the essence of flowers, allowing the vision of various types of flowers—colors, sizes, and levels of complexity—to appear before your mind's eye. You can also visualize a garden abundant with a great variety of flowers.

Out of this radiant diversity, let your subconscious mind bring up a specific flower as the most suitable metaphor for each of the chakras. You may choose the very same flower for all chakras, if that is your subconscious's immediate response to the instructions. You can also envision flowers in the colors that are commonly associated with the individual chakras. Whatever comes naturally to you, follow it uncritically.

Start your visualization by imagining the central column where the chakras reside. Picture it as a straw-like, transparent, flexible, and bluish hollow tube close to the front side of the spine. It starts just below the genitals and pierces through the center of the body all the way to the top of the head.

---

23   https://www.youtube.com/watch?v=W9B0mpxvYms.

Now turn your attention to the lower end of the central chan-nel, the root chakra, which is located deep inside the area of the perineum. Breathe into the area and feel how with each inhalation, you gather the energies within it; with each exhalation, you release it outside the body. In the first chakra, the flower should uniquely face downward, toward the earth, to receive nourishment from the dimension of nature and biological life.

As you breathe into the perineum, let any image of a flower appear in that area, still in a closed state. It may be deep red, the color popularly associated with the root chakra, or any other color. With each exhalation, you are gently urging the flower to gradu-ally unfurl, from deep within the perineum all the way to its exter-nal part, until its petals fully unfold. Allow the wide-open flower to absorb the wisdom of the earth while it releases any tension or trapped energy in the chakra. Its openness implies agreeing to become unconditionally embodied in this life.

Shift your attention to the area behind the pubic bone, where the sacral chakra is centered inside the central channel. Breathe into this deep point within the abdomen: with your inhale, gather energy from this point at the center of the body; with the exhale, release it in an outward direction through the pubic bone. An outward-facing sacral chakra can receive the life force required for enhanced vitality and passion.

As you breathe into the chakra within the center of the body, let any image of a flower appear in that area, still in a closed and shy state. It may be orange, the color popularly associated with the sacral chakra, or any other color. With each exhalation, you are gently urging the flower to gradually unfurl, from deep within the lower abdomen all the way to its external part, until its petals fully unfold. Allow the wide-open flower to absorb life force while it releases any tension or trapped energy in the chakra. Its openness implies agreeing to participate in life's adventure and to fully experience and feel.

Shift your attention to the area behind the solar plexus, where the solar plexus chakra is centered inside the central channel. Breathe into this deep point within the abdomen and sense the sunlike, cosmic powerhouse that is pulsating in it. With the inhale, gather energy from the center behind the solar plexus and with the exhale, release it in an outward direction through the solar plexus. An outward-facing solar plexus chakra can receive the life force required for self-mastery, willpower, and attainment.

As you breathe into the center behind the solar plexus, let any image of a flower appear in that area, still in a closed and shy state. It may be yellow, the color popularly associated with the solar plexus chakra, or any other color. With each exhalation, you are gently urging the flower to gradually unfurl, from deep within the solar plexus area all the way to its external part, until its petals fully unfold. Allow the wide-open flower to absorb life force while it releases any tension or trapped energy in the chakra. Its openness implies willingness to overcome obstacles, contacting your own power and daring to achieve your goals.

Shift your attention to the area behind the lower center of the chest, midway between the two breasts, where the heart chakra is centered inside the central channel. Breathe into this point that is your innermost self; with the inhale, gather energy from the center behind the chest and with the exhale, release it in an outward direction through the lower center of the chest. An outward-facing heart chakra can receive the life force required for the ability to experience love, connectedness, and unity with others and with the world at large.

As you breathe into the area behind the chest, let any image of a flower appear in that area, still in a closed and shy state. It may be green, the color popularly associated with the heart chakra, or any other color. With each exhalation, you are gently urging the flower to gradually unfurl, from deep within the lower chest all the way to its external part, until its petals fully unfold. Allow the wide-open flower to absorb life force while it releases any tension or trapped energy in the chakra. Its openness implies readiness to remove self-defense and to experience trustful intimacy and vulnerability.

Shift your attention to the area behind the Adam's apple, where the throat chakra is centered inside the central channel. Breathe into this deep point within the throat; with the inhale, gather energy from the center of the throat and with the exhale, release it in an outward direction through your Adam's apple. An outward-facing throat chakra can receive the life force required for a free-flowing exchange between your inner world and the external world.

As you breathe into the point behind the Adam's apple, let any image of a flower appear in that area, still in a closed and shy state. It may be blue, the color popularly associated with the throat chakra, or any other color. With each exhalation, you are gently urging the flower to gradually unfurl, from deep within the throat all the way to its external part, until its petals fully unfold. Allow the wide-open flower to absorb life force while it releases any tension or trapped energy in the chakra. Its openness implies willingness to be seen by others and to authentically reveal your innermost self.

Shift your attention to the area behind the brow, midway between the eyebrows, where the third eye chakra is centered within the central channel. Breathe into this deep point within the brain; with the inhale, gather energy from the center of the brain and with the exhale, release it in an outward direction through the brow. An outward-facing third eye chakra can receive the life force required for wisdom, depth, and supreme intelligence.

As you breathe into the point behind the brow, let any image of a flower appear in that area, still in a closed and shy state. It may be purple, the color popularly associated with the third eye chakra, or any other color. With each exhalation, you are gently urging the flower to gradually unfurl, from deep within the brain all the way to its external part, until its petals fully unfold. Allow the wide-open flower to absorb life force while it releases any tension or trapped energy in the chakra. Its openness implies readiness to listen to and receive true knowledge.

Shift your attention to the end point of the column, between your eyebrows and your crown, at a point more toward the back of the head, where the crown chakra is centered inside the central channel. Breathe into this uppermost point inside the brain; with the inhale, gather energy from the depth of the brain and with the exhale, release it in an outward direction through the top of the head. An outward-facing crown chakra can receive the life force required for contacting the source of life and the transcendent dimension of one's being.

As you breathe into the point within the uppermost part of the brain, let any image of a flower appear in that area, still in a closed and shy state. It may be violet or white, the colors popularly associated with the crown chakra, or any other color. It can also be multicolored. With each exhalation, you are gently urging the flower to gradually unfurl, from deep within the top of the head all the way to its external part, until its petals fully unfold. The flower should uniquely face upward, toward the heavens or deep space. Allow the wide-open flower to absorb life force while it releases any tension or trapped energy in the chakra. Its openness implies willingness to remove individual barriers and to immerse one's being in the ocean of pure existence.

Now connect once again with the downward-facing flower of the root chakra, at the area of the perineum, and then contact the crown chakra's upward-facing flower. Supported by the vision of the central channel, feel them like two ends of one stem, or like an unusual flower with two heads. Breathe into the stem, from its lowest point to its uppermost end and the other way around. Do this several times, feeling the full flowering of the garden of your being.

Slowly and gently open your eyes, keeping the sense of open chakras with you for the remainder of your day.

• • • • •

This visualization can also be helpful when you feel that one of your chakras is blocked. Visualizing the blocked chakra turning toward the world, opening up like a flower, is an immediate way to balance it.

Generally, this meditation is a suitable metaphor for the seven-day chakra path: every day you water and cultivate one flower of your seven-layered being, until finally, on Sunday, you come to recognize that this cultivation has naturally led you to a sense of inner completeness. Moreover, in the same way that one chakra day supports and flows into the next, nourishing one chakra naturally invigorates the one that follows. The stem that connects all seven chakra flowers is just like the thread that links all seven chakra days—the thread that we call the week.

MONDAY: ENGAGING THE ROOT CHAKRA ON THE DAY OF GROUNDING

Slightly inside the perineum—between the anus and the scrotum or vulva—the Muladhara chakra resides. The Sanskrit word *moola* means "root" or "foundation," which is precisely what this chakra is all about: as the root of the entire chakra system, it is the foundation of our whole existence, responsible for everything that manifests in the world of form.[24] A solid and flourishing tree must have deep roots that support and nurture it; Monday is your chance to deepen your roots and establish healthy ground for all the week's activities.

---

24   Satyananda, *Kundalini Tantra*, 137–38.

Feel the Day of Grounding

Good morning. You have just woken up to the first day of your week's creation. People tend to rise on their first day with reluctance, experiencing the "Monday blues." Yet, with your new perception of Monday's blessed role in your life, you will beat this feeling and wake up excited. Could you imagine the God of the Old Testament starting his grand seven-day cycle with melancholy and a shrug of resignation? Of course not! This was a day to remember, when the immense potential of creation awaited the guiding hand of a creator who could make something out of nothing.

Today you summon light to illuminate your entire week. Take a deep breath and feel your power. You have the power to structure your life, put it in order, and set in motion a healthy and balanced flow. Just like the creator, you get to design your week's vision. Wake up before everything else infiltrates your world, take a broad look at the week ahead, and begin to prepare the foundation on which it can be optimally realized. Even if your week already seems suffocatingly packed with duties and expectations, imagine that it is an empty canvas on which you are free to rearrange all its different components into one holistic masterpiece.

What do you need to do to make your life a masterpiece? The root chakra is not about grandiose shifts and visions. God, in the sense of the great cosmic design, is in the details—yes, those seemingly nagging, often forgotten details of your life that, when lovingly taken care of, bring about the sense of stability and harmony. That is why the Day of Grounding is devoted to those many details that can improve and balance your life. It is your chance to consider all that could strengthen your foundations, from nutrition to redesigning your house to achieving better time management.

Many of these details have been neglected in favor of other, more pressing engagements or sometimes, simply because they seem like something you cannot be bothered with. But when overlooked for too long, life's smallest details become problems and begin to scream for your attention. Today, be determined to lead your life by patiently, wakefully, and enjoyably paying attention to all those aspects before they need to scream.

It is so much easier to build a rich and fulfilled life on well-established foundations. For instance, when your body is healthy and strong, you have sufficient stamina to face life's challenges, whereas a frail and exhausted body makes any obligation feel utterly tedious and unbearable. This is the secret that the root chakra, the governor of your entire skeleton and spine, discloses to you today: "Begin your week by taking care of me and I shall reward you with the sense that you can safely and confidently put both feet on the ground as you welcome the week ahead."

Recognize the Blessings

As you begin your day, open up to receive its radiant wisdom, gifts, and powers. The Day of Grounding pulls you out of the ethereal dimension of Sunday's pause and places you directly into the world of matter and form. Monday calls you to take care of your earthly stability before anything else. Having appreciated the beauty of timelessness during your weekend, this day teaches you the value of time: time as a gradation through which you construct your life, brick by brick, and rejoice in the steady flourishing that you have achieved.

It is time to face the world. Yet what the root chakra tells you is that you do not have to face it with a feeling of dread, overwhelmed with anxiety, worry, and stress. If you thoroughly follow this day's teaching, it will establish a deep silence within you. Unlike the more known silence of meditation, this relaxation results from the knowing that everything in your life is in place. By intentionally dedicating a full day every week to all the structures that maintain your existence, you can gain more and more of this inner peace. Life feels uncontainable only when you lack an overview of its various dimensions and the steps needed to put each into order. As soon as you attain this mastery, you will be able to flow more easily and freely into the rest of the week.

The Day of Grounding gifts you with the capacity to clear your table. When too many neglected details begin to pile up, your mind too becomes disturbed, messy, and ineffective. Clear your table to clear your mind. As much as possible, relieve yourself of previous obligations, especially those that chase after you for months. Intentionally look for any unresolved business in your material plane. What steps should you take today to promote balance and health in your life? Are there any issues revolving around your body, home, family, community, finances, or workplace? Have you overlooked your unsettled physical, emotional, or mental condition for too long?

Take a caring look at all these matters without the anxious feeling that all must be unraveled today. After all, you will have many more Mondays, and two of the major qualities that your root chakra would like to awaken in you are patience and perseverance. In the material dimension, processes cannot be rushed. In fact, they may often demand a steady cultivation, with cautious attention to the smallest details. This can be a challenge for those who tend to be scattered, jumpy, and even ungrounded. Making your Monday the Day of Grounding is one powerful way to heal this resistance and to develop a more mature understanding of life as a long-term project.

Think for a moment of the tireless passion that drives some insect communities to construct their beehives, anthills, or termite nests. Hating details, like resenting over-complex bureaucratic procedures, will get you nowhere. On the other hand, if you clear one day for this purpose while knowing why you do so, even those seemingly nagging elements become meaningful, an essential ingredient of your week as a whole.

One last blessing of this day is growing your connection with the wisdom of your body. The root chakra is associated with the subtle body of nourishment called *Annamaya Kosha*.[25] As the chakra of basic health, it reminds you to ensure that you are physically nurtured and supported. Be aware of your body's needs, as they are the ingredients that sustain the roots of your being more than any other.

Connect with the Day's Happiness

The Day of Grounding may strike you as far less romantic and exciting than the other six days. It can even seem like a day of mere preparation for the days that follow. This narrow perception can cause you to miss out on the happiness that awaits you today: the happiness of grasping the subtle laws that determine the levels of health, harmony, and peace in your life.

When you control these laws, you attain the exhilarating sense of mastery over your life—a true self-leadership. Put simply, you know how to live in this world of form and action. You

---

25 Satyananda, *Kundalini Tantra*, 140.

are equipped with the knowledge that can help you command processes in the real world. It is like the delight of an amateur gardener who has learned the laws that make flowers bloom, trees grow, and vegetables spring from the earth. The Day of Grounding is for you to become your very own expert gardener.

Mastery means being on top of all of life's aspects. And this mastery starts with the joy of grabbing your planner to create your week. Remember, time can be managed artfully and life is your creative process, a completely shapeable raw material. Instead of staring at your schedule and thinking, *How am I going to do all that?*, comfortably place yourself in the position of a creator. Aim to see everything fall into place and you will quickly realize that time stretches with your creative intent.

The more you relax into this day, the more it will reveal to you its inherent quiet ecstasy. Your determination to create an orderly and supportive environment will release the sense of authentic harmony inside you. This harmony is not limited to your home or office; in the very same way that Chinese feng shui and the sacred architecture of the Hindu vastu shastra harmonize people with their surroundings, it is an alignment with the laws that govern the cosmic order as well. Through it, you tune in to greater cycles of growth and natural evolution. Indeed, in today's context, even ensuring that you have a healthy routine can endow you with the feeling that you are part of a larger order.

Repeat These Affirmations

"Today…

… I bring my body, mind, and entire life to a peaceful balance."

… I am creating the foundations of a healthy and happy week."

… I embrace the small details and put order into my life."

… I give shape and structure to my life."

… I pay full attention to the needs of my body."

… I am learning how to nourish myself."

… I settle into my body as my first home."

… I say yes to life and all its challenges."

… I heal my relationship with life on earth."

… I connect with my inner stability in a world of constant change."

Engage Your Root Chakra

Before anything else, make sure that you say yes to the week's challenges. This internal consent will make you rise on your feet this morning fully embodied. Feel that you are entering Monday with your entire being. If you trace some resistance, look for its origin—this is often an instinctual fear or a certain lack of confidence that starts at the level of the root chakra.

Make a list of the messy aspects of your life that could benefit from your attention. You will be surprised to realize that the more your awareness grows, the more forgotten elements will begin to surface. Then look at your list and choose one messy aspect to focus on today. If this aspect cannot be easily resolved in one day, you can make it your Monday project for several consecutive weeks.

Dedicate time to creating your schedule. Do not rush. Enjoy your creation. Shake off the sense of powerlessness in the face of a long list of commitments. Be determined to prioritize, even if you need to defer some obligations or your own activities. Having the seven-day chakra path as context already makes life much easier since you know where to place each activity and are also encouraged to reserve time for those aspects that are habitually overlooked in your life. However, if you find scheduling tasks overwhelming, look for a book or a course that can teach you the art of time management.

Monday is the day for all the duties and tasks that you do *not* feel like doing. Root chakra activities are often time-consuming and horribly technical. If you are not inclined toward technicalities, take comfort in knowing that it is just a one-day focus. You have Tuesday—the Day of Joy—as your sweet compensation! Make sure that you do not become too rigid in placing all of your practical duties on Monday's schedule. If your doctor is available only on Wednesdays, do not immediately search for another one; just use Monday as the day in which you set up appointments.

If you are the dreamer type who likes to think big yet hates practicalities, define the first or next practical step needed for your project and follow it today. Even if this particular step is not as exciting as your grand vision is, remember that all visions must eventually flow to the root chakra to manifest in the world of form. In general, adopt a practical mode today and do things diligently, making sure that you follow a process to its completion (at least within the limits of the day).

Lovingly take care of your body. Do you have any lingering physical problems? Does your body suffer some chronic pain or discomfort? Are there certain medical procedures that are long overdue? Have you taken the time lately to bring your body to the next level of radiance and high energy? This is your chance not only to act on your body's behalf but also to study your body's wisdom through books, articles, videos, and courses. Learn about toxins that might hinder your health, supplements that can strengthen you, or physical exercises that heal pain.

Fix things! This is a good time to fix not only your body but also your car, furniture, home, and any broken (or nearly broken) devices. You can also develop your handiwork by investing time in some do-it-yourself projects.

Rearrange your house or office. A safe and relaxing environment is crucial for root chakra health. More than that, the root chakra requires cleanliness and orderliness. Monday is a good time to throw away old stuff that has accumulated in your basement, to clean more thoroughly than usual, and to make your house more beautiful.

Practices to Empower Your Day

Activation. Smile into your root chakra or use the chakra flowering meditation in chapter 3 to open it up like a flower toward the earth, feeling the nourishment and support that flow from Mother Nature. Make sure that you let the chakra's healing power spread to the legs and feet and throughout the spine. Alternatively, you can breathe into the perineum slowly and deeply, visualizing that with every breath, you are deepening and thickening the roots of your being. You can also stand up, put both feet firmly on the ground, and, fixing yourself like a robust tree, say yes to your week's journey. If you find it suitable, intone or mentally utter the root chakra's seed mantra, Lam.

Inspiration. Watch or read materials about organization, time management, financial management, cultivating patience and diligence, making lifestyle changes, do-it-yourself ideas, physical health, bodily wisdom, nutrition, diet, healthy recipes, supplements, posture, the wisdom of nature, the communal life of bees, ants, and termites, and so on.

Vision. Feel the previous week that ended and the current week that has just begun. How would you like to build your life from this point onward? How could you creatively structure your week for this purpose? Visualize yourself in a profoundly balanced physical, emotional, and mental state. What does it look like? Examine if there are blockages and resistances that keep you from being able to seriously commit to this day. Finally, decide on one activity and one practice that can bring you closer to a body-mind balance.

Recommended Meditation Practice

We are walking all day long, mostly unconsciously. We move from the living room to the kitchen to grab something to eat. On our way there, there are precious moments that can be used for meditation. By the time you are in front of the fridge, you could already be someone different, a fully present version of yourself. Ordinarily, the purpose of walking is to take you from one place to another. But in walking meditation, the walking there becomes filled with consciousness. You slow down and become one with the movement itself. Of course, this is not done at an ordinary pace, although as soon as you get used to the inner rhythm, you can walk faster and still retain your blissful attention. Through walking meditation, you also learn to put your feet on the ground and to really agree to walk on this earth. In this sense, it can also heal your relationship with Mother Earth. In addition, walking meditation is a preparation for living and acting while being in a state of awareness.

• • • • •

You can do this meditation barefoot or with socks or light shoes on. Start by standing and anchoring yourself. Stand with your feet hip-

width apart and balance your weight evenly on both feet. Take the time to feel the stability of the ground. Bring your awareness to your body, noticing how your body feels as you are standing.

Once you feel rooted, start walking extremely slowly, keeping your eyes lowered on the ground a few steps ahead of you, not looking at anything in particular. Walk back and forth along the same short, straight path. When you reach the end of your path, come to a full stop, turn around, pause, and then start again. If your attention wanders, keep bringing it back to the present moment. Enjoy every step you take. Kiss the earth with your feet, imprinting gratitude and love as you walk. As you walk, mentally repeat, "In the here" with every inhale and "In the now" with every exhale.[26]

Keep your attention on the variety of sensations and perceptions of the present moment. Feel your feet touching the ground, the movement of your muscles, the constant balancing and rebalancing of the body. If at any time you feel like standing still or sitting down to practice, do so.

Pay attention to any areas of stiffness or pain in the body; consciously relax them. Be aware of your location in space, the sounds around you, and the air temperature. Be aware of the beginning, the middle, and the end of your stepping. Become aware of your present emotional state. Notice your state of mind. Is it calm or busy, cloudy or focused? Does your mind rest in the here and now, or is it daydreaming?

After fifteen minutes, relax. Stand and gather all the energy from the practice into your standing. You will notice today that you have plenty of opportunities to continue the practice in a much less formal way while walking from place to place. Even if you don't have a reason to walk, interrupt your activities with just a few minutes

---

26   Nhat Hanh, "Walk like a Buddha."

of movement. Remember: slow down your walking and make it conscious. You will realize that the journey is the purpose, not the getting there.

Other Practices

- Add deep red—the all-sustaining and deeply grounding color of the root chakra—to your clothes, workplace, or home.

- Focus on physical activities that build your stamina and endurance, like long-distance walking or gardening. Choose repetitive, patient physical work. Eat grounding foods such as root vegetables, home-cooked meals, red and orange foods, fermented foods, and warming spices like cardamom and cumin.[27]

- Practice mindfulness. This widespread meditation-in-action connects body and mind and grounds your attention in the action of the present moment. As a result, it is a highly balancing exercise.

- Other suitable practices that originate from Eastern wisdom are mindfulness breathing meditations; Vipassanā meditation, which focuses awareness on breathing and bodily sensations; Jon Kabat-Zinn's body scan; and the qigong standing meditation (*Zhan zhuang*).

- Try visiting a chiropractor, an osteopath, or another practitioner that works with the musculoskeletal system and can align your spine. This has a twofold effect; correcting your posture improves physical health and the flow of life force, and at the same time, it enhances confidence and the feeling

---

27 "Get Grounded and Thrive This Fall."

of being grounded. Qigong—the centuries-old system that coordinates body posture, movement, breathing, and meditation—has a similar effect. Massaging your legs and feet to unravel root chakra tension is also recommended.

- Enjoy some earth meditation—there are many such techniques that can attune you to the earth element and to planet earth.

- Monday is a good time to heal foundational traumas. If you have experienced past shocks concerning sudden changes in life, physical injuries or severe illnesses, accidents, or violence, these are all stored in your root chakra. Look for methods that can help you relieve the instinctual fears and anxieties caused by such memories.

Notice the Challenges

Be aware whether it is time to face certain issues that arise from your Monday encounter with the foundational center of your being.

Examine whether you are confronted with tendencies such as feeling scatterbrained or ungrounded. Look for resistances that you may experience, such as the wish to avoid long-term processes, small but crucial details, or a healthy routine. Pay attention to whether you find yourself struggling with time pressures or a schedule that constantly gets out of hand. Inspect unconscious feelings; perhaps you feel that living on this earth is difficult or even scary. Detect worries and anxieties that may encompass your daily activities. Notice whether your residence fails to provide you with a deep and satisfying sense of home. Pay heed to root chakra–related physical symptoms, especially ongoing muscle pain or tension, such as neck pain or backaches.

You can either contemplate these challenges in writing or look for methods of teaching that guide you on your way to resolving them.

Journal

Have a journal or a notebook on hand to record your thoughts and observations throughout the day. Feel free to take any direction in your writing, but here are some questions you could reflect on in relation to the work you are doing for the root chakra:

- To what degree do I experience a sense of inner stability that remains steady even in the face of change and external turbulence?
- Do I experience worry and anxiety? If so, what insight can I bring to these moments to release such emotions?
- Do I love my body? Can I identify what throws it off-balance and what nurtures and heals it?
- How can I nourish other beings that rely on me, like my children, pets, or plants?
- Do I enjoy creating my schedule, or do I feel constantly overcome by the sense that there is never enough time in the day?
- Do I avoid dealing with necessary technical details?
- How diligent am I when completing processes that require time and patience?

Conclude the Day

This has been your encounter with the first dimension of your being, the dimension of grounding represented by your root chakra.

Express gratitude to this day. Recall what you have done throughout the day, either in terms of practice or intention. Recall events that may have been directly or indirectly associated with the learning of the chakra. Do not attempt to critically evaluate how much you have accomplished today. Even small steps are actual steps that you have taken, and you have certainly managed to stir not only this particular chakra but your entire chakra column toward a greater enlightenment.

Just before you go to sleep, prior to getting into bed or while already lying in it, bring your awareness to your root chakra, deep within the perineum. Visualize that this chakra is superbly active, pulsating and rotating like a wheel that is spinning around its axis, thanks to your devoted attention today. Imagine that at the center of the wheel, there is a concentrated and highly potent point that is glowing with red light.

Feel how this concentrated point of red light begins to spread throughout the body, covering your legs all the way to your feet and extending to the top of your head. Feel how through this visualization, the chakra is releasing its unique consciousness and wisdom into both body and mind. Allow the chakra energy to reach any physical, emotional, or mental blocked area with its healing powers and to unravel and soothe that area through its glowing red light. Now your being as a whole, from head to toe, is radiating with red light; even the surface of your skin is emitting this light.

Encompassed by this red light, contemplate the greatest lesson of the root chakra for a moment: You are able to experience a sense of unconditional and independent stability and security deep inside you, even in the midst of an unstable and endlessly changing world.

Now let the red light dissolve back into the concentrated red point. By dedicating your full attention to one chakra, you are now naturally and effortlessly taking a leap to the next one on the chakra ladder. For a brief moment, feel anticipation for tomorrow's frequency: the sacral chakra's Day of Joy.

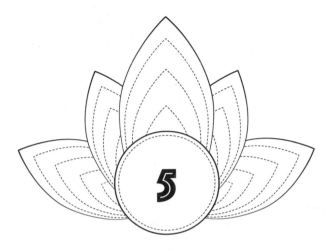

TUESDAY: ENGAGING THE SACRAL CHAKRA ON THE DAY OF JOY

At the lowest point of your abdomen—at the level of the pubic bone, just above the genitals—the sacral chakra (Swadhisthana) resides. The Tantric scriptures speak of it as the repository of our dormant life force, the potent source of all passion.[28] Whereas the traditional worldview treats this chakra as a spiritual barrier that might lead to attachment to sensual temptations and desires, its positive side determines your capacity to fully enjoy and appreciate life's tastes, juices, and pleasures. Tuesday is your opportunity to celebrate the sensual dimension of your life and to color your entire week with the sacral chakra's colorfulness.

---

28   Satyananda, *Kundalini Tantra*, 146–55.

Feel the Day of Joy

Good morning. You have just woken up to a day when your five senses are invited to expand and let in all the possible joys of life. Before anything else, smile. Even if you are still somewhat hazy or full of thoughts, never mind. By letting a wide smile spread on your face, you will contact Tuesday's frequency, informing your sacral chakra that you are game.

Notice how beautifully located this Day of Joy is. Happily sandwiched between the Day of Grounding and the Day of Power, it helps break any excessive sense of linearity and progress. While all three days belong to one phase that is wholly dedicated to the cultivation of your basic relationship with the material world, Tuesday acts as a naughty disruptor, making sure that you do not get stuck in the groove of only focusing on duties, details, and tackling challenges like any adult "should."

Tuesday is a celebration of life itself. In so many ways, the universe is a party of eruptive energies, bodies, and passions. The many interactions between these elements offer countless thrilling and delightful experiences. Tuesday allures you to leave your routine behind and join this party. Your daily commitments and engagements, which are all future-oriented, show you the meaningfulness of a carefully built life. But Tuesday is all about life in the here and now, life's meaning in this moment that generously stretches in all directions.

Shake off your concern that in following the Day of Joy, you might lose precious time required to make sufficient progress this week. First of all, the chakra week offers you three full days to act seriously in the world: Monday, Wednesday, and Friday. Second, progress is endless, and if you suppress that nagging feeling in your lower abdomen that tells you that life cannot be only that, you might end up having all your life's juices and passions dry out. When you were a child, you embodied the knowledge that life in itself is pure joy that requires no justification. You do not need to work hard to deserve it. It is your birthright to enjoy this gift today.

As much as possible, do not rush today; you have enough time to pause and be conscious of life's beauty and the very fact that you are alive. Breathe this simple recognition into your lungs. Then ask yourself what is truly and deeply enjoyable for you. Let enjoyment be your guiding compass today; it connects you to this dimension of your life.

Are you still in bed?

Recognize the Blessings

As you begin your day, open up to receive its radiant wisdom, gifts, and powers. The sacral chakra is the center in you that determines the degree of your excitement about life. How much passion is burning in you to start a new day? A new day is not the equivalent of another day; it is the feeling that the day is an unexplored potential of experiences, revelations, and creativity, not a repetition of what has already been fixed as your routine. Tuesday is all about regaining the sense of exciting freshness. It is your precious opportunity to contact life's flame in you.

Give spontaneity a chance. Pursue impulses and feelings rather than thoughts and concepts. Surprise yourself. At least for today, life does not need to move in straight lines. When did you last consider your day an unpredictable adventure? Often, disrupting routine opens a door to brilliant, out-of-the-box ideas or to solutions for lingering problems that our linear thinking has overlooked as a result of its narrow and fixed perception.

Spontaneity is one way to feed the sacral chakra. Indeed, it is a hunger-stricken center in you, and as you find more ways to satiate it, it will repay you with a restored energy, equipping you with an overflowing life force and releasing any trace of exhaustion or depression. It will fill you with the lost sense of the child that you were, feeling that life is a playground and that you are a player.

But what do malnourished sacral chakras like to eat? Pleasurable impressions and sensory participation in life's delights, from feeding your eyes with beauty and aesthetic pleasure, to allowing your body to experience intimate touch, to the intoxicating sensation of sweet foods and artful cuisine, to laughter that spreads with healing forces throughout your body. There is no need for cautious moderation today. There are enough chakra days to restrict your passions and channel them in more "refined" directions. Today's teaching is to feel more strongly and experience more totally. While it is good to tame some of your self-destructive impulses, make sure that you do not throw the baby out with the bathwater; don't become morally "good" at the expense of your colorful—even wild—parts. Indeed, many addictions and obsessions are twisted forms of this suppression. As soon as you water this chakra, joy reappears in its original and pristine form.

Tuesday's message to you is to activate your body and its senses as extensions of nature's explosive energies. Think of butterflies, rainbows, and spring flowers; all are bursts of life's joy of creativity, generously brushing our vision of the world with intense colors. Your body is not merely a vehicle that leads you from the office to your sofa; it is an inseparable and vibrant part of nature, and through its senses it has the power to explore this life of sights, sounds, tastes, smells, and sensations. Follow the elementary powers of your senses to literally get in touch with life's many offerings.

Connect with the Day's Happiness

There are two major types of meaning and happiness. One is found in the way we steadily build a stable life that, at the same time, keeps growing and expanding. This sense of an unfolding realization of our potential is deeply connected with the feeling that there is a future to aspire for. But this is only half of the picture. The other type of happiness cannot derive from the future. In fact, it can be known only by rejecting even the subtlest form of waiting. This is the happiness of the here and now.

The happiness of now reveals itself when you do not rush to participate in the grand project of the future. Instead, slow down and look around. Rest your attention upon the simpler, mostly overlooked realities of life. For instance, that you are alive and breathing, or that the clouds create breathtaking formations against the background of the vast blue sky, or that the happy and sweet voices of playing children infiltrate your office. Indeed, if you take a deep look into the heart of the moment, you realize that it is problem-free. It transcends the subconscious obsession with searching for problems and struggling to resolve them. At the core of the now there is a bubbling, gushing sense of joy, and from it, the cosmos spreads with its immensely artful expressions. Acknowledging all that, you may realize that you hardly contain the riches of this moment, so how can you possibly yearn for anything more besides it?

Seek this type of happiness today. And, as an expression of it, engage yourself as much as possible in activities that are driven by passion and that are not measured by their outcome. Do things for no good reason: paint, write a poem, stroll in the park, or take pictures that capture minor details of life and the world. Not all actions should be purposeful, intended for achieving another cause; some things just happen, out of sheer impulse, and disappear without leaving a trace.

Pleasures are a good example of activities that arise from the happiness of the now. They appear and disappear. Dancing with totality is meaningless; you will not be able to retain that ecstasy, so what is the point? There is no point. Pleasure is meaningful only in the now. Therefore, enjoy pleasurable experiences and know that you cannot keep them. Experience them deeply; they hold unknown depths of feeling and sensation. There is so much to discover in the realm of feeling, yet only your deep devotion to the now can let you into this kingdom.

Repeat These Affirmations

"Today…

… I am following my enjoyment instinct."

… I release the joyful child in me that only wants to experience and explore."

… I allow the force of spontaneity to show me the way."

… I acknowledge life's beauty in the here and now."

… I am becoming aware of the celebration of nature and the cosmos."

… I am noticing life's bright colors."

… I am opening all my five senses."

… I am feeling the river of life force gushing inside my body."

… I am dancing my way through life."

… I keep my inner smile no matter what happens."

Engage Your Sacral Chakra

Make enough space for leisure and even allow yourself to be lazy. This may strike you as an odd "activity" since it is, in many ways, a non-activity. Yet, feeling that you have breathing space in the middle of the week disrupts the sense of continuity and nourishes the sacral chakra.

Be playful—and not only in spirit. You can even clear some time for gathering with good family or friends and be wholly dedicated to playing games together. Games of any kind entice your inner child to come out. Connecting to children and animals may be another way to easily access playfulness.

Be creative for no good reason. (Creativity that has a clear purpose of manifestation and self-fulfillment belongs to Friday, the Day of Expression.) Today is the day to write a poem or a short story, paint, sing, or redesign your house, all for the simple reason of sheer delight. The sacral chakra's creativity is a joyful expression of being alive and stirred by overflowing feelings.

Find ways to enjoy the various arts. You can visit a museum or attend a theatre show or musical performance. Wash your eyes and ears with beauty that evokes your aesthetic appreciation. Merge with music that you dearly love. Spending time in nature can fill you with the marvel of creation as well.

Go on an adventure. Adventure is not necessarily a tremendous or extreme journey. It can be an unplanned experience that breaks any of your daily habits. For instance, taking the car and driving an unfamiliar route, turning the order of your scheduled events upside down, or going to surprising events—such as visiting an awe-inspiring planetarium show—can reassure you that there are still new things to discover in life. Even *planning* a vacation or an exciting project can be stimulating: the second chakra is where all exhilarating ideas and visions are first ignited by life's flame.

Take risks. Not all risks are highly dangerous. Actually, many of them simply require your daring to follow them: going on a date; collaborating on a creative venture; initiating a conversation about a subject you would ordinarily avoid discussing; or investing time, energy, and perhaps a little money in a project that would not necessarily be successful. Even while being challenged in life, you can experiment with types of reactions that you would not naturally express. In general, practice going with the flow. Whatever life brings to you, accept it lightheartedly and seek more creative ways to respond.

Cook or bake. Find creative, artful, and delicious recipes. An inseparable part of life's joy is measured by our taste buds. The sacral chakra is particularly inclined to intensely rich spices and intoxicating desserts. Use this opportunity to indulge in a happy dinner with friends or experience some new flavors in an unusual restaurant. Eating with your hands has been proven to be not only a healthy habit that promotes fullness and satiety but also enjoyment.[29]

Be sensual. Your body's sensory contact with the world is a source of many possible pleasures. Receive a massage or enjoy deeply rewarding sexuality. Other satisfying ways to be sensual include cultivating your physical beauty and going to a dance party.

Look for opportunities to laugh as much as possible, like watching a great comedy. Laughter is the sacral chakra's healthy approach to life.

---

29   Rana, "Eating Food with Hands."

Practices to Empower Your Day

Activation. Smile into your sacral chakra or use the chakra flowering meditation in chapter 3 to open it up like a flower toward the world. Alternatively, you can celebrate the beginning of your Day of Joy by doing some dynamic meditation, dancing to music that makes you happy, or taking a quick walk outside to greet the waking world while immersing yourself in the here and now.

Inspiration. Watch or read materials about the power of smiling and laughter, children and the (positive) inner child, the power of imagination, how to remain young in spirit, the arts, beauty and aesthetics, poetry, creativity, the power of colors, nature and animals, healthy sexuality, ecstatic dance, creative cooking and baking, and so on.

Vision. Consider how you could connect more deeply with the joy of life during your Tuesday. Visualize yourself in a state of profound exuberance and enjoyment today. What does it look like? Examine if there are blockages that keep you from fully enjoying your life and your physicality. Is there anything that makes you feel unable to smile and laugh, incapable of suspending all your problems? What are the thoughts that keep you in a serious state this morning? Finally, decide on one activity and one practice that can color your day.

Recommended Meditation Practice

Laughter has been proven to help decrease anxiety, stress, and depression, so it makes a lot of sense that it has been made into a widespread, deliberate meditation.[30] Laughter meditation is a way

---

30   Eisler, "Laughter Meditation."

to tap into joy that will flow into other parts of your life. It helps you maintain the perspective that there is still much to be thankful for and to celebrate in your life. Because laughter meditation is not tied to something actually being funny, you create a link to noncausal joy. You connect with your authentic laughter, which has no reason or rational explanation. This meditation invites you to set aside your serious adult self; it is difficult to laugh and think at the same time. Laughter meditation is also an opportunity to access your emotions in a creative way. When you're focusing on laughing, you're concentrating on the release of a major emotion, which can open the door to other major emotions like sadness, anger, and fear. Laughter releases trapped energy into the surface, and in this way it enables energy to flow. Sometimes it can turn into crying—that's perfectly fine! If this happens, you can allow it for a moment until it becomes laughter again.

• • • • •

The main focus of this meditation is, of course, to laugh. There are no objects to concentrate on or visualizations to take you elsewhere. Start by relaxing your body through some movement. Stretch your arms high above your head, rock your body side-to-side, massage your jaw, and yawn at least two times to loosen your mouth and relax the jaw muscles. Next, find a comfortable position to sit or stand. For some, lying down may relax the stomach muscles and allow laughter to flow more easily. Follow your intuition.

Close your eyes and contact the inner laughter that awaits you at the depth of your being or think of something funny. Start by slightly smiling and then begin laughing without too much effort. From giggling, gradually move to deep belly laughs. Try different types of laughs to encourage your true laugh to come through.

Even if it begins as a forced feeling, the forced laughter will catalyze authentic laughter in no time—follow it until it becomes natural.

As you progress, lose yourself in laughter. Be possessed by the laughter. Let it drown everything in you, all thought, all emotion. Let all boundaries between you and existence disappear. Allow it to melt away all tensions. Let your body roll about in a light, playful way. At times, you may come up against blockages, like anger; laugh them out. Let laughter flood all that is preventing your ecstasy. Do this for at least fifteen minutes.

Then sit or lie on the floor in stillness. Gather all the energy within and be mindful of what comes up for you. You can connect with your lower belly, where your sacral chakra is, by breathing into it and holding it. Purified from laughter and silence, open yourself to a day of laughter. Whenever possible, giggle or even laugh, as if laughing from a joke. Laugh when you feel that you're becoming too serious or forgetting yourself in some unconscious thought or emotion. Remember, if you can laugh now, without a reason, you are free.

Other Practices

- Add vibrant orange—the sacral chakra's color of joy—to your clothes, workplace, or home.

- When selecting a suitable physical exercise for your Day of Joy, make sure that it is a fun type of exercise rather than one that focuses on achievement.

- Breathing exercises, such as the various yogic pranayama and full yogic breath, can promote a fuller breathing—and a fuller breathing implies an enhanced life force.

- Any type of dynamic meditation suits the Day of Joy. The underlying principle of such meditations is that the physical release leads to spiritual elevation. In addition, they liberate the body from mental inhibitions and allow the life force to flow more freely. Try one of Osho's active meditations, such as his dynamic meditation, Kundalini meditation, Nataraj, or Gourishankar. Osho was a twentieth-century Indian mystic who believed that people should engage in cathartic meditations prior to a quiet, inactive sitting meditation.[31]

• There are several Eastern practices that enhance the life force and awaken the dormant potential of the sacral chakra. A few examples are the Chinese tai chi, Mantak Chia's Taoist tantra and inner smile, the Tibetan tummo (inner fire) meditation, and any type of yogic Kundalini practice. Follow them in moderation—remember, the sacral chakra does not respond to goal-oriented actions.

• Forest bathing, or shinrin-yoku, is a Japanese practice that employs the powers of forests and trees for healing processes. The practice, which is all about connecting to the forest through the senses, is quite simple, yet its proven health and spiritual benefits are enormous.[32]

• Experiment with shamanic or spiritual events that are intended to lead participants to trancelike states. Often this is done through manipulation of the breathing or musical journeys.

• As much as possible, surprise yourself with different practices every Tuesday. The sacral chakra is not fond of repetition!

---

31   Osho, *Meditation*.
32   Li, "'Forest Bathing' Is Great for Your Health."

Notice the Challenges

Be aware whether it is time to face certain issues that arise from your Tuesday encounter with the sensory center of your being.

Do you find it hard to allow yourself a day full of joy? Do you feel that it is a waste of time or something that you do not deserve to experience? See if this day confronts you with moral issues or rigid concepts of the "correct" way to live that nest deep inside you. Consider whether your experience of pleasure is limited because you are too afraid of being disappointed when life's pains strike again. Look for a tendency in you to push down urges and impulses in a way that suffocates your life force. Be aware of any sense of depression—the dark side of the sacral chakra—that is lurking at the background of your being, keeping you from truly engaging joy. Pay attention to whether this day brings up issues of complicated or conflicted sexuality. Notice if you are confronted with certain addictions and obsessions—twisted forms of joy—that you have developed over time.

You can either contemplate these challenges in writing or look for methods of teaching that guide you on your way to resolving them.

Journal

Have a journal or a notebook on hand to record your thoughts and observations throughout the day. Feel free to take any direction in your writing, but here are some questions you could reflect on in relation to the work you are doing for the sacral chakra:

- To what degree do I experience a sense of inner joy even when daily routine threatens to erode it?

- Do I succumb to feelings of depression? Am I often overcome by exhaustion and lifelessness? If this happens frequently, what insight can I bring to these moments?
- Can I identify the thoughts that rob me of my intrinsic joy?
- How much pleasure am I capable of experiencing?
- Do I try to avoid pain so often that I end up experiencing very little of life?
- Is my bodily freedom inhibited by taboos and shame? How can I release my body into its natural freedom?
- Can I identify some addictions of mine? How can I transform them into healthier patterns that really make me happy?
- Do I feel capable of smiling right now for absolutely no reason, or even bursting into laughter?
- Do I breathe fully at the moment?
- Do I feel playful, imaginative, and adventurous?
- Do I feel connected to nature? What can I learn from nature about my own way of life, physicality, and sense of aliveness?
- What is my relationship with sexuality and how can I take it to the next level?
- What experiences fill me with beauty and awe?

Conclude the Day

This has been your encounter with the second dimension of your being, the dimension of joy represented by your sacral chakra.

Express gratitude to this day. Recall what you have done throughout the day, either in terms of practice or intention.

Recall events that may have been directly or indirectly associated with the learning of the chakra. Do not attempt to critically evaluate how much you have accomplished today. Even small steps are actual steps that you have taken, and you have certainly managed to stir not only this particular chakra but your entire chakra column toward a greater enlightenment.

Just before you go to sleep, prior to getting into bed or while already lying in it, bring your awareness to your sacral chakra, behind the pubic bone. Visualize that this chakra is superbly active, pulsating and rotating like a wheel that is spinning around its axis, thanks to your devoted attention today. Imagine that at the center of the wheel, there is a concentrated and highly potent point that is glowing with orange light.

Feel how this concentrated point of orange light begins to spread throughout the body, covering your legs all the way to your feet and extending to the top of your head. Feel how through this visualization, the chakra is releasing its unique consciousness and wisdom into both body and mind. Allow the chakra energy to reach any physical, emotional, or mental blocked area with its healing powers and to unravel and soothe it through its glowing orange light. Now your being as a whole, from head to toe, is radiating with orange light; even the surface of your skin is emitting this light.

Encompassed by this orange light, contemplate for a moment the greatest learning of the sacral chakra: You are able to experience a sense of unconditional and independent joy and happiness deep inside you, even in the midst of life's two opposites, pleasure and pain.

Now let the orange light dissolve back into the concentrated orange point. By dedicating your full attention to one chakra, you are now naturally and effortlessly taking a leap to the next one on the chakra ladder. For a brief moment, feel anticipation for tomorrow's frequency: the solar plexus chakra's Day of Power.

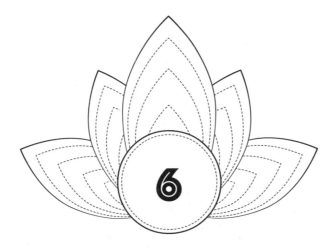

WEDNESDAY: ENGAGING THE SOLAR PLEXUS CHAKRA ON THE DAY OF POWER

The Manipura chakra is located in the center of the torso above the navel, where the solar plexus is situated as well—hence, it is commonly known as the solar plexus chakra. Manipura is often compared to the dazzling heat and power of the sun. Similarly, this subtle center is the source of the fire and heat that propel our dynamism, willpower, and ambition. When deficient, we hardly find motivation or commitment and shy away from challenges that pull us out of our comfort zone. Wednesday is your opportunity to tap into this hidden treasure that empowers you to take your life into your own hands.

Feel the Day of Power

Good morning. You have just woken up to a day when the hero inside you will take the lead. While Tuesday's sweet taste is still in your mouth, feel the surge of heated energy, like an ignited engine, in the pit of your abdomen. There is no doubt that life is to be celebrated for its inherent beauty and creativity, but what about the heights you could reach if you gathered forces and dared to want more?

It is time to raise your head to locate and define your own mountain peaks. Your solar plexus chakra tells you that it is not enough to experience life at ground level and to fulfill the same duties and commitments every day. Life is also a ladder of growth and success; with every step, you overcome limitations and expand your being. What would you consider an achievement today? What is your next step on the ladder?

Your idea of achievement may not necessarily be career-oriented. There are many ways of self-realization, and only you can determine what your success story should include. This day is more about clarifying and gathering your willpower, deciding that you are not giving up on your goals even if that requires battling with your inner enemies or seemingly insurmountable external obstacles. What really counts is the effort you make to build your inner powers and the way you discipline and harness your being until it turns into a well-targeted arrow. Becoming a hero is, before anything else, learning to govern the forces within and transcending elements that drag you down, such as laziness, fear, and weakness.

It is not always easy to know what you want. You may find out that your true desires are buried beneath thick layers of suppression, self-denial, and fear. Wednesday encourages you to dare to dream; what do you want? What are the necessary first steps on your way to fulfillment? Declare your desires and remain loyal to them, even if the road is full of pitfalls and overshadowed by the dread of failure. The pitfalls are there to sharpen your will even more; eventually you will be immune from pressure.

It is this sense of indestructible self that the Day of Power strives to consolidate in you: an inner immovability that remains unshaken even in the face of the harshest challenges. Think of it as an energetic immune system, the growing capacity to contain life's pressures and to experience yourself bigger than them. To achieve this highest of goals, you are called to strengthen your individuality and presence. Equipped with true inner power, you can finally gain an unfailing and authentic self-confidence.

Recognize the Blessings

As you begin your day, open up to receive its radiant wisdom, gifts, and powers. This day empowers you to shift from a state of scattered energy and lack of mental focus into a fully integrated being. People are often torn between different and even contradictory wills and voices, each pulling in another direction. When you know the one thing that you want more than anything else, you become a unified, directed, and magnetic presence in the world.

Another important teaching is Wednesday's call to move from a passive and submissive approach to being a co-creator that actively participates in the shaping of reality. Life's play is not only about responding to whatever comes your way; without your proactive steps, the dance is not complete. If certain past experiences have caused you to feel too small to willfully influence the stream of life, this is your opportunity to defy those ghosts that tell you what you can and cannot do. Remember that the sense of helplessness and worthlessness is just one more element to overcome on your way to true inner power.

Use this day to come into contact with the depths of your potential. Unleash the Achiever in you and you will quickly realize that the higher you aspire and the more daring you become, the more you actually push the boundaries of potential. Skills and abilities you have never known will become available to you. Make sure that the goals you define are not limited by hidden assumptions that you will fail or reach too far.

One more Wednesday gift is acquiring the power of self-discipline. This quality has nothing to do with social pressures and expectations. It is a recognition of your own dignity and nobility that arises from deep within. To achieve substantial success, you cannot afford to shirk effort and committed action. Even to be able to follow this seven-day path, you ought to remain faithful to the inspiring inner call that ignited your determination. Now it is up to you to generate momentum for this new positive habit. Self-discipline is a loyal servant of your strongest will; it is the concentrated energy required to push beyond your familiar, lazy patterns.

Guided by today's blessing, recognize also the unbreakable element at the core of your being—the solar plexus chakra. This center contains the dormant capacity to function as an ever-radiating sun that cannot be diminished, even in the face of crisis and failure. Indeed, used wisely, much-dreaded moments of weakening only help to fortify its immaculate presence.

Connect with the Day's Happiness

The unique happiness of the third chakra lies, first and foremost, in liberating your will from its cage. While everyone has desires, it is considered somewhat immoral to admit them fully, even to oneself; being "good" is associated with wanting less. However, willfulness is not an egotistical part of you that you should be embarrassed by. Suppressing this healthy force drains your natural vitality. If anything, the problem is not that you want too much, but that you do not want strongly and clearly enough. As soon as you release your will, you become synchronized with the pulse of the cosmos, like plugging your solar plexus into its source of unending energy.

Wednesday's happiness is also deeply connected with the sense of having a future, something that is worth looking for. While Monday is all about the delight of feeling solid and strong foundations and Tuesday reveals the happiness of the here and now, Wednesday is the time to recognize the other half of the picture: the elevation that fills you as you are progressing toward a longed-for mountain peak with your entire being. In fact, even defining goals can be uplifting, including goals that you might not necessarily be able to achieve or destinations that will eventually be replaced with more realistic or accurate ones.

The experience of achievement contains two types of fulfillment: the journey toward your holy grail and the moment in which you finally hold it in your hands. Many successful people have come to realize that their greatest excitement lies in the unwavering determination with which they remove any obstacles in their path. Much of the sense of triumph takes place already then, when it is still unclear whether the goal is achievable or not.

Start today by defining and visualizing the victories you wish to attain in any aspect of your life—in your spiritual progress, personal relationships, health, or creativity—and see for yourself how your pulse quickens and your energy level is heightened. Moreover, sense the joy that fills you whenever you defeat fears and other external and internal weakening voices. In each of us there is a warrior that strives to come out victorious—the warrior that is aroused as a dormant memory when we watch or read heroic legends and mythologies.

The deepest aspect of this warrior spirit is its ability to be invincible. Paradoxically, being invincible is not the result of fighting really hard, but the outcome of a silent presence that remains unaffected under all circumstances. Each day is filled with encouraging and weakening incidents; even our fluctuating thoughts and feelings create changing impressions of distress and optimism within us. When you develop an equilibrium of presence in yourself, one that is shaken by neither positive nor negative events, you finally become the master of your own happiness.

Repeat These Affirmations

"Today…

…I gather all the forces of my being to follow what I want."

…I shamelessly reveal and declare what I want."

…I am taking one more step toward my highest goals."

…I find the power in me to overcome any obstacle."

…I overcome my inner enemies."

…I contact my inner power regardless of life's ups and downs."

…I have the power to contain life's pressures and demands."

…I am the hero of my own life."

… I learn how to say no when needed."
… I contact my sense of self-dignity."

Engage Your Solar Plexus Chakra

Set and declare your goals. Start by creating a list of ten goals for the next five years, this year, or simply this month. Do not limit yourself to topics like your career and finances; think more broadly of how you could take each aspect of your life to the next level. (Make sure that you avoid abstract, intangible goals like "I want to be happy.") Then, ask yourself which goal is the one you want to achieve the most and declare it to yourself. Clearly define the steps you can take now to get closer to your ten goals. Bear in mind that at least some action should be taken this week; do not let a week go by without achieving an actual breakthrough.

Challenge yourself. The Day of Power encourages you to strain your capacities and to move beyond your limits. Since our brain's automatic tendency is the pursuit of pleasure and the avoidance of pain, it will signal "That is too much!" whenever you defy your current limits.[33] Whereas Tuesday was all about effortlessness and the celebration of life, push yourself today to replace the instant gratification of pleasure with the satisfaction of overcoming. Choose a mountain to climb—this can be an actual mountain if you have one around, an effortful physical activity like experimenting with higher-level exercises or running, acquiring a new skill, learning a new language, waking up earlier than usual, or entering a more intense spiritual practice. Be patient: sooner or later, you will get your second wind!

---

33   Fernando, Murray, and Milton, "The Amygdala."

Drop a bad habit. If you have accepted a negative or even self-destructive habit (such as overusing your smartphone or overeating) only because you feel too weak to resist it, this is the time to come out victorious in the battle. You may not overcome it for good, but at least start the process of disassociating from it. Even abstaining from this habit for a day is a small victory that becomes registered in your mind as a new possibility. Seek out some good advice in books or videos if you feel that you need to be empowered to break your habit.

Finish tasks. We often begin something, despair, and leave some loose ends to be tied up the next day (which might not happen). Today, persist with taxing actions and do not abandon them until they are successfully completed.

Achieve more than usual. If you often think, *This is it—this is my maximum capacity; if I do more, I'll burn myself out*, experiment today with overcoming exhaustion and making your full day even fuller. There is no need to worry about depleting your energy reserves, since it is only one day a week, a day enveloped by two far softer days.

Aspire for excellence. Try to *really* do your best on Wednesday. Excellence is a noble quality of the solar plexus chakra, and it is a form of accomplishment in itself. Refuse to settle for less than the ultimate fulfillment of your skills and talents. Gather your energy, heart, and mind to devote your full attention to the smallest details that make your work a masterpiece.

Face and contain moments of weakness. There are disappointing incidents of small defeats, hurts, and frustrations each day. Our brain's immediate tendency is to avoid the pain involved as much as possible. Instead, welcome these moments, knowing that by testing your courage, certainty, and resolution, they can help you solidify and crystallize your authentic presence in the world.

Practices to Empower Your Day

Activation. Smile into your solar plexus chakra or use the chakra flowering meditation in chapter 3 to broadly open it up like a flower toward the world. (I recommend visualizing the solar plexus chakra as a sunflower.) Continue your activation by imagining that within your solar plexus there is a yellow sun blazing with the fire of life. Feel how your entire presence emerges from the heated energy of this sun. If you prefer a more active start to the day, chant the solar plexus mantra, Ram, with your attention centered on the upper belly, or try tribal dancing.

Inspiration. Watch or read materials about inner power, ambition, willpower and setting goals, knowing what you want, coaching, focus and concentration, courage and confidence, how to discipline inner energies and forces, overcoming laziness, the quality of excellence, the inner warrior, decision-making, self-mastery, how to get rid of bad habits, success stories, great heroes of past and present, traditions of noble warriors (such as the samurai or the Shaolin monks), motivational speakers, and so on.

Vision. Get in touch with your willpower and all that you hope to achieve. Visualize yourself walking and acting today with a fully integrated presence and a radiating inner power. What does it feel like? Consider fears and insecurities that hinder your willfulness and keep you from achieving your goals. What are your inner enemies? What limitations do you wish to overcome today? Decide on one action and one practice that will enhance your sense of individual power and capability.

Recommended Meditation Practice

In this adaptation of the mountain meditation by Jon Kabat-Zinn, you meditate on the image of a mountain, identifying with it until you become one with it. The nature of mountains is elemental—rock hard—and so they represent immovability, an extension of our core being. Mountains reflect to us what it truly means when we take our seat for meditation. Choose a mountain whose form speaks to you and contact the universal quality of mountainness through it, beyond any particular shape or form. During this meditation, it is recommended to sit in an immovable but not rigid position. By sitting immovably, you use your body as a reminder of the unchanging part in you, the center which is stable and immovable. Realize that the body can sit like that for hours; what "needs" to move is your thought, not your body.

• • • • •

Close your eyes and sit with your back straight. Allow your head to be gently held on your shoulders, keep your shoulders relaxed, and place your hands on your knees. Make sure that you sit in a comfortable position—a position you can hold for quite some time. The only movement you should allow is breathing and swallowing, but even this can be gentle and conscious.

Feel the contrast between your running thoughts and your own choice of immovable position. Let this physical stillness influence your mental stillness. As you allow the body to be still, feel the sense of dignity, resolve, and completeness, whole in this very moment.

Now picture the most beautiful mountain that you've ever seen or can imagine. Hold the image. Let it come into better focus. Observe its shape and its points of contact with the earth and the sky. Notice how massive it is, how solid, how unmoving. Notice how its base is rooted in the earth's crust. Just sit and breathe with the image of the mountain, noticing its qualities.

Bring the mountain into your own body so the image and your body become one. You share the massiveness and the stillness of the mountain. You become the mountain, rooted in this sitting posture, your head a lofty peak, your shoulders and arms the sides of the mountain, your legs the solid base rooted to the chair. With each breath, you become more of a breathing mountain, unwavering in your stillness—a centered, rooted, unmoving presence.

Like the mountain, embody this unwavering stillness when faced with change. Realize that as a mountain you can also add a sort of an inner smile of knowing, like a soft Buddha smile: the smile of knowing that whatever happens, there is this unchangeable, unaffected center in you. Notice how now, as the mountain, your thoughts feel external, more like birds flying around your mountain form.

After at least fifteen minutes, breathe the presence of the mountain into the body and the mind and gently come out of the meditation. Hold the image and feeling of the mountain whenever you can. Bring it up in front of your mind's eye and feel how this presence is affecting your own presence. Remember to do this at times of emotional distress, tension, or challenge. How would you respond to a difficult situation from this mountain-like state?

Other Practices

- Add sunny yellow—the solar plexus's color of intensity and life-enhancing energy—to your clothes, workplace, or home.

- Be stimulated by spicy foods that enhance your fire element.

- Dance to the sounds of tribal music or tribal drums. This African-inspired power dance can quickly arouse the warrior in you and fill your body with the energy you require to confront life's challenges.

- If you are a yoga practitioner, choose more intense and physically straining asanas or more demanding styles like Ashtanga yoga. Add the heat-inducing pranayama Breath of Fire.

- Learn the exercises of the Dutch extreme athlete Wim Hof. Hof, "The Iceman," is known for his ability to withstand freezing temperatures. The method he developed helps people build solar plexus chakra resilience in different ways, from breathing exercises to taking ice-cold showers.[34]

- Engage in any type of martial arts. Such practices are focused on developing the hara—the area behind the umbilicus, which is where the "sea of qi" (vital force) is said to spring from.

- Try concentration techniques. Strengthening your power of attention can train your mind to focus your willpower on one thing.

---

34 Hedegaard, "Key to a Healthy Life."

• Choose meditation practices that enhance your sense of self-presence. Essentially, all meditations help to establish an immovable center in you, so you may also regard your usual practice in today's context and intention. You can use Gurdjieff's technique of self-remembering, or simply center your attention on the basic feeling of "I am" as an ongoing meditation, even while are engaged in other activities. Whenever possible, move your sense of self-existence from the head, the mental center, to the solar plexus, the presence center. When your "I am" shifts to the solar plexus, it becomes real—a truly integrated presence that includes a genuine feeling of existence and vibration. Each time you connect this thought with a deep feeling in the solar plexus, you are enhancing and deepening your sense of presence.

• Practice the "eternal seesaw." This is a highly effective technique that can help you establish inner power: Take a notebook and create two columns. Title one "Moments of Power" and the other "Moments of Weakness." Whenever you have an elevating experience throughout the day, including encouraging thoughts, mention it briefly in the "Moments of Power" column. Do the same with weakening events and feelings. At the end of the day, carefully read these summaries of constant, seesaw-like ups and downs. Consider them as one eternal movement instead of two opposing experiences. Then close your eyes and ask yourself, "Who am I outside this entire game?" There you will find your indestructible self.

• Activate the solar plexus to prevent and overcome disease. As your energetic immune system, the third chakra can play a major role in repelling and expelling psychosomatic disorders and illnesses.[35] If you face some unstable physical condition, even simple and brief forms of activation can awaken this chakra's ability to defeat disease. Breathing into the navel, for instance, sends the vital forces of Manipura up to the brain. Smiling into the chakra or visualizing its flowering toward the world does pretty much the same. A mental way of achieving this effect is by adopting the affirmation "I am fully able to contain this challenge" whenever you are faced with an overwhelming and pressuring situation that might turn into physical distress.

- Heal your wounded will. If you can identify certain traumatic experiences that damaged your willpower and led you to adopt a victim mentality, face them through a deep therapeutic process. Your determination to overcome these memories is already a declaration of true inner power.

- Dare to try firewalking. This practice of walking barefoot over a bed of hot embers or stones originates from ancient India and is considered a test of strength and courage. Of course, this should only be done responsibly, under guidance and within the framework of a seminar.

Notice the Challenges

Be aware whether it is time to face certain issues that arise from your Wednesday encounter with the will center of your being.

As you sit down to define your list of goals, notice if nothing comes up. See if you identify a paralyzing fear of failure that

---

35   Satyananda, *Kundalini Tantra*, 161.

makes you avoid fulfilling your wishes even before taking the first step. Investigate the feeling that you could never really be the ambitious type. Examine whether you feel overcome by laziness and distraction as soon as you meet the first obstacle on a new journey. Look for issues of dependency and authority in your life that make it difficult for you to settle in your own inner power. Become aware of strong and influential personalities around you whose goals and destinations always seem more important than yours. Pay attention to whether you tend to explode with anger whenever life does not give you exactly what you want, when you want it.

You can either contemplate these challenges in writing or look for methods of teaching that guide you on your way to resolving them.

Journal

Have a journal or a notebook on hand to record your thoughts and observations throughout the day. Feel free to take any direction in your writing, but here are some questions you could reflect on in relation to the work you are doing for the solar plexus chakra:

- To what degree do I experience a sense of inner power even in the face of events that seem to weaken me?
- Do I experience powerlessness often? If so, what insight can I bring to these moments?
- How do I cope when I feel humiliated?
- Do I constantly compare myself to other, more successful people?

- How do I manage my anger and the anger of others?
- Do I feel that I am capable of drawing the line, saying "no," and resisting pressure?
- Do I feel capable of challenging myself and stretching my capabilities?
- Do I dare to define goals and to pursue them with determination?
- Do I know what I want? Have I declared it clearly to myself and to others?

Conclude the Day

This has been your encounter with the third dimension of your being, the dimension of power represented by your solar plexus chakra.

Express gratitude to this day. Recall what you have done throughout the day, either in terms of practice or intention. Recall events that may have been directly or indirectly associated with the learning of the chakra. Do not attempt to critically evaluate how much you have accomplished today. Even small steps are actual steps that you have taken, and you have certainly managed to stir not only this particular chakra but your entire chakra column toward a greater enlightenment.

Just before you go to sleep, prior to getting into bed or while already lying in it, bring your awareness to your solar plexus chakra. Visualize that this chakra is superbly active, pulsating and rotating like a wheel that is spinning around its axis, thanks to your devoted attention today. Imagine that at the center of the wheel, there is a concentrated and highly potent point that is glowing with yellow light.

Feel how this concentrated point of yellow light begins to spread throughout the body, covering your legs all the way to your feet and extending to the top of your head. Feel how through this visualization, the chakra is releasing its unique consciousness and wisdom into both body and mind. Allow the chakra energy to reach any physical, emotional, or mental blocked area with its healing powers and to unravel and soothe it through its glowing yellow light. Now your being as a whole, from head to toe, is radiating with yellow light; even the surface of your skin is emitting this light.

Encompassed by this yellow light, contemplate the greatest lesson of the solar plexus chakra for a moment: You are able to experience a sense of unconditional and independent power deep inside you, even while facing life's eternal seesaw of ups and downs.

Now let the yellow light dissolve back into the concentrated yellow point. By dedicating your full attention to one chakra, you are now naturally and effortlessly taking a leap to the next one on the chakra ladder. For a brief moment, feel anticipation for tomorrow's frequency: the heart chakra's Day of Love.

THURSDAY: ENGAGING THE HEART CHAKRA ON THE DAY OF LOVE

At the core of your chakra system, right at the bottom of your sternum, Anahata, the heart chakra, abides. It is the seat of your personal love and emotional life as well as the potential source of universal, unlimited love.[36] The heart chakra is greatly dedicated to the healing and fulfillment of the entire range of your relationships—not only with all others but also with yourself. When its work is done, it feels unbreakably whole and free to give unconditionally. Thursday is your opportunity to nurture your world of relationships and to dare to practice the full opening of your heart.

---

36   Satyananda, *Kundalini Tantra*, 169–71.

Feel the Day of Love

Good morning. You have just woken up to a day that is wholly dedicated to the expansion of your heart. As you open your eyes, feel it throbbing within your chest, not only the physical organ but also the subtler element that is the carrier of your deepest emotions—the part that can open and sometimes break, love and sometimes shrivel.

Perhaps contacting and expanding the heart comes naturally to you—in this case, your day is going to be an effortless celebration of your heart's most authentic desires. If you are less tuned in to the heart's rhythm, the Day of Love is a significant phase of your week: a chance to ensure that this precious dimension of life does not get lost in everyday hustle and bustle. In both cases, you may discover that the heart rapidly responds to your attention, nearly bursting forth, since it forever awaits your call patiently and compassionately.

This softening pause in the midst of the week—which perfectly divides the week's first and second halves—is particularly vital after fiery Wednesday and with the completion of the earthly material phase. On the solid ground of your now-awakened three lower chakras, it is time to take a broad and kind look at the world around you—not through your ordinary, physical eyes, but through your heart's eyes. Equipped with the profound sensitivity of the heart, turn your gaze to notice and acknowledge the existence of those around you who may, explicitly or unknowingly, require your care and warmth. This includes your very own being, which could be in some sort of emotional starvation.

Today you are invited to take the time to take care: feel yourself and others, attend to their unanswered needs, heal them with your love, embrace their sorrow, and make them smile through words and gestures. Use Monday's time-management skills to schedule opportunities to intimately meet your loved ones—partners, children, friends—on Thursdays. Look into their eyes, cherish their existence, rekindle your love; aren't you blessed to have them around? Is this shared path obvious at all?

It is also a time to notice broken relationships. Have you allowed a connection to wither or a conflict to build up? Use your Thursday to throw a healing light on past wounds and emotional traumas. Purify the heart from bitter memories and renew your trust in yourself, fellow humans, and the world at large.

Remember that healing does not necessarily end in your personal relationships. The heart tells us that all beings of this world exist in a web of unbreakable interconnectedness. Thus, today's practice of loving kindness and compassion can also be directed toward suffering humans, animals, and plants and toward our decaying planet. Open your heart's ears to hear the cry of those in need; could your heart be extended to include them in your Day of Love?

Recognize the Blessings

As you begin your day, open up to receive its radiant wisdom, gifts, and powers. Its first message to you is simple yet striking: if you have passed an entire week with your heart empty, none of what you have done truly matters. On the surface, you may have excelled in completing tasks and meeting goals, but the acute hollowness within your chest might make you wonder what this ceaseless action was all about.

This is because the heart is the one element in you that is most strongly associated with the meaning of life. This meaning is not something you might ever know, but you can definitely *feel* when it is absent. On the contrary, when your life is filled with love—love of what you do and love in the relationships with those around you—such doubts rarely arise. Thursday is your time to consciously declare why you do what you do and to imbue your week with this undeniable fragrance.

Use this time to unravel the emotions stored within your heart chakra and to melt away its hardening as a result of the week's disappointments. You are encouraged to listen to your emotional condition, to sincerely ask, "How do I feel?" Whatever is reflected in this day's mirror of compassion, you can channel and transform it through sincerity and technique.

If your sensitivity to your loved ones has been eroded by life's demands or accumulated bitterness and anger, this day can support you in the rehabilitation of your damaged connections. It is always wise to nourish a relationship instead of only treating it in times of crisis. Seek out ways to responsibly clear away toxic thoughts and feelings that overshadow your emotional exchange. If you neglect to do that, you might end up feeling lonely even when you are surrounded by family and friends. Thursday allows you to strengthen your connections and to enjoy the clear feedback that echoes the effort you have invested. Moreover, as soon as your heart begins recognizing those on the planet who are suffering, your empathy and action can finally dissolve the sense of being cut off from the web of interconnectedness.

Thursday reminds you that your heart is bigger than you think. It can give love *today*, exactly as you are, not only after you have treated it and healed it completely. Humanity's greatest teachers have told us throughout history that in giving, there is the most meaningful receiving. This is exactly what your heart, your greatest teacher, invites you to try today.

Connect with the Day's Happiness

What the Day of Love offers you is the bliss of intimacy. When hearts get to connect—through an embrace, a deep look of recognition, words of appreciation, or a vulnerable sharing—they overflow and open. To enable instances of true intimacy, reject the false signals of stress that warn you that there can never be enough time for such events. These are the moments that as we grow old, we wish we could have had. Relax and breathe together in a timeless zone; listen to one another without much emphasis on your own judgments and opinions, and look for the common ground that has always attracted you to one another.

The deepest wish of the heart chakra is to open unreservedly. We are, however, mentally conditioned to believe that a closed heart is a protected heart. Ironically, this strategy only enhances our suspicion and oversensitivity. Experiment today with the very opposite direction, total abandonment of your heart's wall, and you are likely to find that by forgiving and being willing to experience pain, you feel stronger. Anyone at the end of a profound healing session who has agreed to remove their protective layers and to allow their heart to once again shine forth has tasted the joy of the open heart. If you are steeped in emotional pain, look for transformative methods to make this miracle happen.

An integral element of the heart's happiness lies in its capacity to help us to come out of ourselves and become givers, even to those outside of our immediate circle. We all know the thrill of surprising someone with a gift or a heartwarming gesture. While our conditioned thought often focuses our attention on our own neediness and sense of lack, fulfilling others' needs and hopes and witnessing our ability to elevate people's lives is a gateway to our own sense of completeness. The Dalai Lama put it eloquently: "If you want others to be happy, practice compassion. If you want to be happy, practice compassion."[37]

Another dimension of happiness can be revealed to you today by seeking to define the intention and meaning behind your activities and goals. Your heart is happy when it has the right motivation, and its motivation is always connected to service for others or to a creative passion; both are forms of love. Sometimes simply adding the intention "I do this because I love" will suffice to place your action within the context of your heart's one true reason.

Repeat These Affirmations

"Today...

... I perceive the world through the eyes of my heart."

... I accept myself and all others through the sweetness of my heart."

... I disregard imperfections and only see wholeness."

... I aspire to make others happy."

... I do everything out of love."

... it is my turn to love."

... I open myself to universal love."

... I rest inside the inner cave of my heart."

... I realize the power of the vulnerable heart."

... I open my heart unconditionally, even when it hurts."

---

37   Dalai Lama and Cutler, *The Art of Happiness.*

Engage Your Heart Chakra

Get in touch with your feelings. Emotions can be unknowingly suppressed because they interfere with efficient functioning during the day. Use your Thursday to feel your feelings. As much as possible, be sincere. Is there any sense of lack or an unanswered yearning? If this lack or yearning is directed toward someone, it may remain unfulfillable. Look for methods that can satisfy and channel these feelings more constructively, such as strengthening your self-acceptance and emotional independence.

Take care of yourself lovingly. What gestures of self-love could you make today? Perhaps you feel reluctant to embrace yourself, feeling that for some reason you do not deserve it. Yet, when you nurture yourself, you may already start feeling more comfortable with your body and mind. One way to find out what your being truly requires is by asking, "If I fully loved and forgave myself, what would I do today?"

Detect one or more existing relationships in your life that you can improve on the Day of Love. Is there any connection that you have not supported lately with your parents, your partner, children, friends, dog or cat, or even the dying plants in your house?

Make time to meet your loved ones. Make sure it is not constrained by other duties and that your smartphone is put aside. Be present and attentive. Bestow more physical warmth and emotional sensitivity on them.

If you feel lonely, be proactive and seek out ways to join warmhearted circles and gatherings or one-on-one interactions. Set your intention to make new friends. And do not despair—remember that there are nearly eight billion people on this planet, many of them yearning for deep connections just like you.

Focus on what you can do for others. Begin by thinking of someone in your surrounding area that seems to need help. Is there one thing that you could do to elevate someone's spirit today?

Support activism. Open your heart to more global forms of suffering. While becoming conscious of the overwhelming degree of suffering in this world might dishearten you at first, you must not conclude that your contributions are futile. There are people whose vocation in life is to serve as activists in different fields. Even if you do not hear such a calling, you can empower those who do. Donating to charities, signing petitions, learning about the small steps that you can take in your own life to make a stand, or even publishing posts that can draw people's attention to a higher cause are all good ways to fulfill your heart's wish to alleviate suffering.

Volunteer. This does not have to be the classical form of volunteering; whatever you do that is not money-oriented and that will give you nothing besides heart fulfilment falls into this category. If your work permits it, you can perhaps reserve a time slot on Thursdays for unpaid service.

Practices to Empower Your Day

Activation. Smile into your heart chakra or use the chakra flowering meditation in chapter 3 to broadly open it up like a flower facing the world. Take a long moment to cherish close or remote people whom you love. Feel how your heart is connected to them as if by a thread, forming a web of connectivity. Visualize that your heart is linked to other beings by the very same thread, in ever-distancing circles, until you find yourself connected to all that is. Alternatively, use the recommended meditation practice of headlessness or select any of the following heart practices to activate compassion and abundance.

Inspiration. Watch or read materials about love, compassion, forgiveness, balancing and opening the heart chakra, nonviolent communication, the power of togetherness, self-healing, self-acceptance, mending broken relationships, devotion and sacrifice, selflessness, activism, volunteering, things we can do for the planet and animals, inspirational figures who have demonstrated the power of love and sacrifice, and so on.

Vision. Consider all your opportunities of love today. How can you strengthen this thread of connectivity, attention, and care? Are there small or big ways in which you could enrich your activities with the presence of love? Visualize yourself walking in the world with an unconditionally open heart, imbuing your day with deep emotional awareness. What does it look like? Examine if there are blockages and resistances that keep you from expressing this love. Finally, decide on one activity and one practice that will awaken your heart's qualities and capacities.

Recommended Meditation Practice

Headlessness is a simple, direct, and physical way to draw energy from the head to the heart and to awaken your heart center. We wrongly identify the center of our being as the head, but the head is actually meant to be the heart's servant. You can make this transition physically. By imagining and feeling that you are headless, you can literally move down from the head into the heart.

As soon as you do that, your entire perception becomes clear and complete. At the beginning it will be only "as if," but slowly you will settle in the heart. Headlessness can actually make you feel like you are really moving to the heart for the first time and settling there.

• • • • •

Sit comfortably, but don't slouch. Do not close or lock your chest. Allow your shoulders to fall gently backward so that your entire chest area feels open and spacious, as if you were presenting it to the world. Imagine that you have lost your head, as if instead of your physical head there is now purely space.

When you feel that you are headless, your center of gravity naturally flows to your heart. It's like an effortless falling down of your center. Breathe gently into the chest area, feeling more and more that this is where you are. From your new location in the chest, the brain, eyes, ears, and mouth are mere tools rather than who you are. Try to feel how your central vision is located in the chest area, like a pair of hidden eyes. Through these eyes, you are actually looking at the world inside and outside you. What happens when you look out at everything from here? What are the qualities of vision and listening that belong to this area? How are they different from your usual sight and hearing? Does this shift to the chest relax anything? Does it make your vision more sweet, compassionate, or forgiving? This way of looking will change your total personality and pattern because whatever the heart looks at, it sees from the angle of wholeness, harmony, and peace.

Try to look at a particular challenge or conflict in your relationships from your new "head." How do you see this issue now, from the perspective of your heart? How do you perceive others from this space? How do you see life in general? With each breath, feel how the chest expands at the expense of the head area and opens up even more. The wider it gets, the more the head area is consumed by it. As your new head, what does your heart know today? Is there anything—even just one thing—that it knows deeply, beyond any doubt? Declare it.

After at least fifteen minutes, take one more deep breath and slowly and gradually come out of the meditation. As you open your eyes, retain the sense of an open chest and outward flow. Prepare yourself for a headless day! Walk around as headless as possible. Look at everything from your chest, and don't forget to also look at yourself through the heart's forgiving eyes.

Other Practices

- Add deep green—the all-nourishing color of the heart chakra—to your clothes, workplace, or home.

- Relax into a hug. If you have a willing relative or friend, a hugging meditation can be very soothing: relax your entire being into each other's arms, allowing it to satiate your emotional needs and soothe any stored pain.

- Read books or watch movies based on true stories that exhibit the greatness of the human heart. Examples include *Gandhi* (1982), *Schindler's List* (1993), *Hotel Rwanda* (2004), *Selma* (2014), and *A Beautiful Day in the Neighborhood* (2019). It is significant to be inspired by people like you and me who have shown incredible powers of devotion and selflessness.

- Send or email appreciation letters. Taking the time to acknowledge someone's beauty, virtues, and talents is an event that instantly widens both individuals' hearts. Why wait for a birthday or other special occasion? You have Thursdays, and there are many people to embrace with your warm words that are left unspoken.

- Meditate on your merits and others' positive traits. Create a list of all your good qualities and beautiful attributes. This is not an ego list; on the contrary, it is the human tendency to notice our shortcomings and limitations that derives from a fixed mental habit. You can also sit with your friend, child, partner, or colleague and form lists of each other's gifts, capacities, and talents, one column for each of you. Emphasize qualities one of you naturally has that the other doesn't. Then create a third column that combines all these capacities—all the good qualities that your connection contains from both your personalities. Realize that together you have formed a greater entity blessed with many qualities and capacities! Considering your combined energies and gifts can be very empowering.

- Practice love as the motivation for all your actions. Use the affirmation "I do it because I love" before even your most mundane activities, such as washing the dishes and driving your child to school. This declared motivation adds an immediate depth of meaning to the action.

- Practice nonviolent thought and action for a day. During your Thursday, refrain as much as possible from judgment, anger, and arguments. If critical thoughts and emotions arise, center your being in the chest area and look at your subject of criticism through your heart's eyes.

- Try the Buddhist loving kindness meditation (Mettā meditation), compassion meditation (Karuna meditation), or the giving and taking meditation (Tonglen meditation). Such forms of practice enable you to enhance empathy and appreciation.

• Practice heart opening. There are many heart chakra opening techniques, including music meditations and visualizations. Look for the relatively unknown Tibetan Buddhist meditation called "The Inner Cave," which is a particularly powerful form of heart chakra opening. Its power lies in the ability to lead you to the innermost layer of your heart, which has remained unaffected by any of your difficult emotional experiences.

• Heal and be healed energetically. There are simple methods of healing one another by laying one's hands on the body and transmitting positivity and love.

• Try crying meditation. Similar to Tuesday's laughter meditation, the heart stores many unshed tears; releasing them can purify and lighten the heart. You can follow the second phase of Osho's Mystic Rose Meditation, or simply put on some music, trace a point of unresolved sadness in you or recall some past hurt, and allow that feeling to start a cathartic process.

• Forgive someone. Forgiveness is one of the easiest ways to open the heart. It is made possible when you remember that it is, before anything else, your very own liberation from the past as well as an expression of power rather than weakness. Write a letter of forgiveness to a person, but do not feel compelled to send it; simply use it to propel a process of release from your haunting memories.

- Heal emotional shocks and past disappointments. You can do this by turning to a form of guided therapy or by applying a self-guided technique.

- Engage in devotional practices such as sacred singing or prayer. The sense of devoting your life to a greater reality is an instant heart-opener. You can also chant the heart chakra seed mantra, Yam.

Notice the Challenges

Be aware whether it is time to face certain issues that arise from your Thursday encounter with the emotional center of your being.

Pay attention to whether you experience emotional dependency and attachment that leaves you powerless and fearful. Consider whether you think of yourself as overemotional or hypersensitive. Notice if it's hard for you to accept yourself as you are, believing that you must earn your very own self-love. Inquire into your inability to forgive and to leave behind past hurts. Explore the possible feeling that there is such a profound sense of lack that you cannot find any capacity to share or give. Examine whether the Day of Love feels like a stranger to you, challenging you to tap into a world that feels unexciting or threatening. Consider whether the habit of judgment and expectation has become too intense to allow your heart to accept others.

You can either contemplate these challenges in writing or look for methods of teaching that guide you on your way to resolving them.

Journal

Have a journal or a notebook on hand to record your thoughts and observations throughout the day. Feel free to take any direction in your writing, but here are some questions you could reflect on in relation to the work you are doing for the heart chakra:

- To what degree do I experience the ability to express love to my dear ones?
- Am I open to receiving their love as well?
- Do I know how to seize opportunities of intimacy, even in the midst of a hectic day?
- Am I capable of selfless and compassionate acts?
- What is friendship to me? Do I follow my own idea of friendship?
- Do I find pleasure in serving others and giving them what they need or hope for?
- Have I reached a sufficient self-acceptance, the ability to feel comfortable with myself and unjudged in my own heart and mind?
- How do I cope with loss, abandonment, or disappointment? If I feel such moments are unbearable, what insight can I bring to these feelings to make my heart stronger?
- Do I know how to distinguish destructive emotions from constructive emotions? What are my strategies for transforming the destructive ones?

Conclude the Day

This has been your encounter with the fourth dimension of your being, the dimension of love represented by your heart chakra.

Express gratitude to this day. Recall what you have done throughout the day, either in terms of practice or intention. Recall events that may have been directly or indirectly associated with the learning of the chakra. Do not attempt to critically evaluate how much you have accomplished today. Even small steps are actual steps that you have taken, and you have certainly managed to stir not only this particular chakra but your entire chakra column toward a greater enlightenment.

Just before you go to sleep, prior to getting into bed or while already lying in it, bring your awareness to your heart chakra, behind the bottom of your sternum. Visualize that this chakra is superbly active, pulsating and rotating like a wheel that is spinning around its axis, thanks to your devoted attention today. Imagine that at the center of the wheel, there is a concentrated and highly potent point that is glowing with green light.

Feel how this concentrated point of green light begins to spread throughout the body, covering your legs all the way to your feet and extending to the top of your head. Feel how through this visualization, the chakra is releasing its unique consciousness and wisdom into both body and mind. Allow the chakra energy to reach any physical, emotional, or mental blocked area with its healing powers and to unravel and soothe it through its glowing green light. Now your being as a whole, from head to toe, is radiating with green light; even the surface of your skin is emitting this light.

Encompassed by this green light, contemplate the greatest lesson of the heart chakra for a moment: You are able to experience an unconditional and independent sense of love and openheartedness deep inside you, even in the midst of life's emotional disappointments.

Now let the green light dissolve back into the concentrated green point. By dedicating your full attention to one chakra, you are now naturally and effortlessly taking a leap to the next one on the chakra ladder. For a brief moment, feel anticipation for tomorrow's frequency: the throat chakra's Day of Expression.

FRIDAY: ENGAGING THE THROAT CHAKRA ON THE DAY OF EXPRESSION

At the base of your throat, directly behind the thyroid gland, the throat chakra (Vishuddhi) resides. Imagine this chakra as a doorway standing between your inner world and the outer world. The door can be wide open to receive others' thoughts and transmissions from the outer world and to allow the expression of your innermost truths and feelings, or the door can be sealed, keeping your true voice stuck in the throat and your being unrealized and invisible. Friday is your weekly opportunity to activate the chakra of primal sound in order to start expressing yourself courageously and authentically.

Feel the Day of Expression

Good morning. You have just woken up to a day during which you are going to make yourself visible in the world. Yesterday was wholly dedicated to contacting your heart; now it is time to present its beauty and wisdom to the world. Deep down, you know that you have experienced, learned, and realized more than enough to share your being with others. Keeping it to yourself is like caging the bird of your soul, but all it really wants is to sing its song for everyone to hear.

Feel the tingle of excitement down your throat. As long as you hide yourself behind the throat's door, all your true feelings, cherished beliefs, and precious gifts remain unrecognized. Do not leave your throat chakra to suffocate. End its frustration by closing the gap between the way you experience your inner self and what actually comes out of your mouth. Remember the throat chakra wisdom that what has not become a tangible manifest reality does not exist at all, to some extent.

The Day of Expression is an opportunity to pinpoint the truest feelings and most intimate truths and ideals that wish to flow and surface from within your being. The form they will eventually take is not limited to verbal communication. The throat chakra can bring out your authentic being in manifold ways, like music, painting, dancing, and even simply the way you look and present yourself. The latter is highly significant because in your presentation, your entire process of manifestation begins. Become conscious of the way you generally appear and express yourself. Do you take enough space to show yourself in your fullest charismatic potential? What is the experience of others when they meet you? Are you present enough to leave a deep impression on them? With the power of your throat chakra active today, you can freely give rise to a radiating presence in the world.

Since this is a day that encourages your manifesting powers, ask yourself if there is something you believe in and care about enough that you wish to spread its message. Is there anything your experiences and insights have taught you that can help and inspire others? Today is the ideal time to open your ears and listen to your own message. As soon as you get hold of this message, it becomes your vocation; you are called to give it a voice and to ensure that it leaves its mark in the world around you.

And there is more: Friday is an invitation to take an honest look at a long-buried dream or a suppressed grand vision. Can you dare to be that visionary once again? The world is packed with dreamers who have either followed their vision with totality or had to greatly overcome their own fears and hesitations to succeed. Make sure that you surround yourself with such figures who can inspire you to take a first or next step on your way to realizing this dormant potential.

One key to Friday's fulfillment is to place your expression in the context of serving others. Rather than focusing on yourself as the source of expression and inspiration, consider how your skills and abilities could be of use to those around you. Whether you are an artist, an educator, a speaker, or a family member, think of yourself as one who strives to set an example for others to follow.

Recognize the Blessings

As you begin your day, open up to receive its radiant wisdom, gifts, and powers. Friday's first blessing is its capacity to get you in touch with important feelings and thoughts you should release into the world. Of course, no one is supposed to express aloud all that is hidden inside them; some words and gestures should be left unspoken to avoid damaging ourselves or others. There are, however, certain suppressed expressions that suffocate your throat chakra. Allow this chakra wisdom to filter out the unnecessary, leaving you only with the essentials that can help you grow into a fully authentic being.

If you have ever felt the frustration of not speaking your words as clearly as your thoughts do, today you are encouraged to work on clarifying your expression. If others constantly leave you with the feedback that they are not sure what you mean, or if you feel that your interactions achieve the opposite of what you were hoping to achieve, let the throat chakra guide you to acquire new communication skills. Perhaps certain emotional hindrances, such as fear of rejection or a feeling of smallness, will come to light along the way to be recognized and healed.

This very same smallness is challenged even more strongly by Friday because of its capacity to extricate your inner dreamer. Today is not the day to shirk and postpone your wildest visions; compromises can be made afterward, when the inevitable encounter with reality's limitations will test your enthusiasm. But first, dream: now is the perfect moment to close your eyes and let a future greatness emerge from the field of endless possibilities. Every meaningful manifestation starts with the seed of the future, which may seem overwhelming and unreachable at first. Yet Friday is practical enough to require that you take a realistic step toward this grandness.

As a part of dreaming big, the Day of Expression frees you to be an uncynical idealist. We all have a hunch about possible pathways that our community and society could take toward a better future; we hear a cry within us in the face of certain forms of injustice. Our throat chakra is fulfilled when it protests and partakes in world rectification. Empowered by yesterday's awakening of the heart, see if you can become a leading voice rather than a quiet observer.

Connect with the Day's Happiness

There is great joy in manifestation. Think of a child who plants some seeds in the ground and, after a while, finds that one of them has grown into a young tree. Think of an author who catches a fleeting and elusive idea, toils to transform it into a novel, and then gets to witness the exhilaration of its readers. This shift from possibility into actuality is one of life's greatest passions—a passion you can encounter within your own throat chakra by bridging the realm of inner potential and the visible world. *You* are also a seed full of possibilities that aspires to become a tree. Friday is when you water and cultivate the soil so you can become all the richness that you sense inside.

Another aspect of today's happiness is the feeling of alignment, when you manage to express yourself exactly as you feel. Imagine the thrill of a film director who has succeeded in fully translating a complex vision into a living reality on set. In the same way, achieving a lucid and effective statement of your truest feelings implies that you have made it to the real world. If your throat chakra is stuck, the outer world may seem like a stranger. Breaking this barrier brings about the joyful recognition that this is *your* world. You can be your honest self in the world and settle in its midst without needing to fear it or hide away from it.

More happy moments are in store for you if you faithfully follow this day; namely, the satisfaction of being able to affect someone's life, when all the knowledge and skill you have accumulated transforms someone's mind or heart. Influence is how we serve as a part of the greater whole. Just as we are positively affected by others' wisdom, so too we are fulfilled by passing our own talents along the chain of interconnectedness.

But what if our words or deeds are met with indifference, or even scorn? Here the fifth chakra tells us that it is sufficient to express what you have to express, regardless of the way people respond. It is the very wish to leave an impact in the world that matters, less so the consequence. You must not force others to listen; sing your song and let the world and your fate determine the level of applause you will receive in return.

Repeat These Affirmations

"Today…

… I am making my inner light and beauty visible in the world."

… I am allowing my natural expression to reverberate in the universe."

… I am spreading positive influence in the world."

… I am going to change others' lives."

… I dare to be heard."

… I am going to sing the song that I am hearing inside."

… I share what I know."

… I am creating new and unexpected channels of communication."

… I am opening myself to new visions."

… I am listening to my wildest dreams."

Engage Your Throat Chakra

Share an honest talk with your partner, family, friends, colleagues, or boss. Are there feelings and truths that must be expressed even at the risk of conflict? Make sure your words have a constructive intention behind them—otherwise it would be wiser to treat such emotions or complaints through transformative self-practice. Do not demand that others accept what you have to say; remember the law of nonviolent communication that your feelings are, after all, your responsibility. One more way to practice honesty is by daring to say "no," marking your limits despite the inconvenience involved.

Write an article, blog post, social media post, or newsletter about things that matter. We live in the era of the throat chakra, and the virtual world is packed with endless possibilities of self-expression. If you can give lectures, webinars, or YouTube talks on Fridays, this could be another good way to activate the chakra on its designated day.

Devote time to creating or improving your website or other communication channels. Ask yourself if they truly reflect who you are and what you are driven to share. Strive to make them more communicative, sharpen and simplify their statements, and seek out ways to widen your potential audience.

Expand your network. Search for like-minded people through online communities or gatherings where people influence and inspire one another. This is also a great way to practice your communication skills.

Dedicate your Fridays to work meetings and creative brainstorming. While engaging in such discussions, learn to listen to others' opinions, including (and especially) the ones that oppose yours. Remember that the throat chakra is also concerned with receiving others' voices. The findings of cognitive research confirm this essential truth: to make better choices, decision makers should imagine the voices of present gossipers and future critics.[38]

Improve self-presentation. There are plenty of good ways to develop charisma and magnetism and to become a more skilled communicator. Be more conscious of your posture, tone of voice, and clothing style. Do they express what you wish to be or become? Examine your level of spontaneity, clarity of expression, and listening capacity. Record yourself giving a talk and attempting to explain something to others or to yourself and then watch it carefully, analyze your body language and clarity of explanation, and correct accordingly.

Acquire leadership skills to strengthen your ability to influence others. Ask yourself honestly: "Am I setting an example? Do I live what I preach, and do I preach what I live?"

Protest or engage in a world change movement that fights injustice. Because the throat chakra is the chakra of justice, look for a way to be a social warrior in the name of a cause you strongly identify with.

Practices to Empower Your Day

Activation. Smile into your throat chakra or use the chakra flowering meditation in chapter 3 to broadly open it up like a flower toward the world. Feel how you are opening the door of your being through the throat chakra and how your innermost thoughts flow freely until you break the communication barrier. If you prefer a more active start to the day, you can sing, chant, or hum.

---

38   Kahneman, *Thinking, Fast and Slow*, 418.

Inspiration. Watch or read materials about self-expression, effective communication, honesty, spontaneity, nonviolent communication, learning to say no, facing criticism, positive influence, vocation, charisma, leadership, being a visionary, the power of manifestation, creating a vision, decision-making, writing and speech skills, using your voice, figures who embody free expression and powerful manifestation, and so on.

Vision. Get in touch with all the things you could manifest using your inner knowing, creative powers, and skills. What do you care about enough to propel you toward committed action? Visualize how you manifest your best self in the world today, uninhibitedly expressing yourself in real-life situations. What does that look like? Is there anything that suffocates your throat chakra and yearns to come out? Decide on one action and one practice today that can enhance your expression in the world.

Recommended Meditation Practice

Aum is probably the most widespread mantra in the world. It is considered the vibration of the cosmic motor, the divine mantra that keeps bringing the universe into existence. It is the mantra of manifestation and actualization, the first word—this is why some use it for enhanced power of manifestation. Meditators can hear aum resounding in the depths of their meditation because it is not a man-made mantra, but a fundamental sound that has always been there.

Aum is a combination of three basic sounds: A-U-M. (It is not the simplistic form of "om," as it is commonly spelled.) All sounds are said to be made of these three basic sounds.[39] To pronounce the word correctly, open your mouth and say "A" (ahhh). In the same breath, gently close your mouth and the sound will become "U"; close your mouth and the sound becomes "M." These are three consecutive sounds that are basically one long sound, uttered as one. All three sounds should be equally uttered. The utterance should be with a deep, low voice, as if coming from the depths.

• • • • •

Start by intoning, "Aum," loudly and outwardly for five to ten minutes. Intone it slowly and deeply, feeling that you become the sound as much as possible. Let it vibrate through the body, mind, and nervous system, and feel that your entire being is filled with it, every cell vibrating with it.

Then, stop intoning aum aloud and start intoning it inwardly—but still "loudly," so to speak, so the sound spreads all over your body and reaches every part of it. Feel as if your body is a musical instrument and this is the harmonious melody it needs the most. Do this for another five to ten minutes.

Let the sound shift to your subconscious and make it your eternal background—an essential sound that has always been there since the beginning of time, prior to your existence, as if you are only finding it inside. You are no longer chanting it. This is not your mantra. It is the universe's mantra. You are just listening. It exists outside of you, outside of your mind. You are only experiencing its reflection in your mind. Let the sound be long and slow.

---

39   Osho, *Meditation*, 147.

Don't allow yourself to fall asleep; chanting can make you fall asleep because it is mechanically relaxing. Follow each aum as if you were holding it by the tail. It is like a magical creature that can take you to where it came from: the origin of the universe. It emerges from this source and returns to it over and over again. With every appearance, it creates the universe and sustains it, then returns to emptiness. Thus, creation is flickering constantly.

When you follow the aum to its root, let it lead you to the unfathomable depths of the silence from which it emerged. At the end, remain still for a long moment.

Today, allow the aum to resonate slowly in the background. Whatever you look at today now has the eternal background of aum. Let the aum be an underlying sound—even beneath your mundane thoughts and emotions—and you will realize how easily your entire life becomes permeated by profound silence and the effortless state of meditation.[40]

Other Practices

- Add blue—the throat chakra's color of clarity, truth, and trustworthiness—to your clothes, workplace, or home. You can also visualize a blue sky or vast airy space expanding within the throat.

- Empower yourself with affirmations. The throat chakra wisdom includes the materializing power of the word and, before anything else, the words we tell ourselves in the form of unconscious and conscious thoughts. The healing and centering energy of affirmations guide the tone of

---

40 This meditation was inspired by Osho's *Meditation* and Satyananda's *Kundalini Tantra*, both excellent resources.

your inner voice. You can use traditional mantras or the affirmations offered in this chapter, or you can be creative and invent sentences and statements that instantly affect your mindset. Let them be central thoughts today; place affirming reminders around the house.

- Use associative writing to unravel your clogged throat and to find your inner truth. It may be that after years of suppression and self-control, you have lost spontaneity and the natural flow of interaction. Associative writing (or speaking) is a powerful tool that helps you lose control, relieve the feeling of being stuck, and tap into the true voice that glows within you. Sit comfortably with a pen and paper or a Word document and release your confused thoughts and feelings. (Alternatively, you can record yourself talking.) Don't worry about punctuation, grammar, or spelling mistakes, and don't pause to articulate your thoughts. If you have nothing to say, write, "I have nothing to say ..." until the flow is resumed. You can focus on a certain question or conflict that occupies your mind today. For the most part, this practice simply offers a release, yet sometimes, when among the many thoughts a bright and wise thought is spilled out, it yields an unexpected insight. A similar practice is gibberish meditation, when you use incomprehensible talking to clear your mind and throat.

- Sing, chant, or hum. Self-expression can start with a verbal or creative communication; making sounds, beautiful or cathartic, clears out your throat chakra to prepare you for interaction. Enjoy singing, chanting, or humming, either alone or in a circle. Try Osho's Tibetan-inspired Nadabrahma or his Chakra Sounds meditation, which purifies all seven chakras. More intense forms of this practice are screaming (preferably in the context of a group dynamic meditation), intentional laughter (see Tuesday's practices in chapter 5), or crying (see Thursday's practices in chapter 7).

- Discover the harmonizing powers of the Taoist Six Healing Sounds. This ancient technique makes use of six sounds to transform negative energy stored in the organs into healing light.

- Practice "right speech." Right speech (*samma vaca*) has been cultivated in Buddhism. It trains the throat chakra to be balanced and accurate. Each day we give voice to many unnecessary thoughts and feelings—and worse, to some aggressive and hateful elements in us. Such expressions engender disharmony in ourselves and in our surroundings. Violent words are often considered less "wrong" than violent actions, and that is why online comments are often wildly destructive. Some may even think that negative words are justified at times. Yet negativity pollutes your heart and mind and prevents you from realizing the true role of expression: enhancing the positive evolution of yourself and others. At least on Fridays, abstain from lies and manipulations; avoid slandering others; resist rude, impolite, or abusive language; and refrain from indulging in idle talk or gossip.

- Create a vision board. Vision boards are a highly relevant Friday practice to awaken your manifesting powers. Start by closing your eyes and entering a deep state of relaxation. From it, allow a vision of yourself blossoming in a certain field (relationships, career, physical health, etc.) in three, four, or five years. What would ultimate fulfillment of this area of your life look like? In a sense, this vision is not something you mentally produce; think of it as a potential that awaits you in the field of endless possibilities. Do not be content with general or abstract descriptions; make it as detailed as possible and write it all down. Then look for photos and images online that capture the different stages of your vision and assemble it all on a board or in an album, intertwining images and the corresponding parts of your written vision. Focus on it every Friday to feel inspired, but revise the vision board from time to time. On each Day of Expression, define your next steps in light of the board.

Notice the Challenges

Be aware whether it is time to face certain issues that arise from your Friday encounter with the communicative center of your being.

Do you fear that revealing some suppressed parts of yourself might threaten the image you have cultivated? Do you worry that showing your truest self will lead to social rejection? Pay attention to whether you depend so much on people's reactions that you end up saying only what you hope others want to hear. Notice if you feel paralyzed when standing in the limelight or when you have the opportunity to present yourself or your vision. Look for any hindering thoughts and feelings when you find yourself struggling to put your ideas in writing. Do you have a cynical voice inside you that tells you that you have nothing significant to contribute to interactions and discussions? Think of an experience you may have had a painful disconnect between your dreams and the ability to take practical steps toward their fulfillment.

You can either contemplate these challenges in writing or look for methods of teaching that guide you on your way to resolving them.

Journal

Have a journal or a notebook on hand to record your thoughts and observations throughout the day. Feel free to take any direction in your writing, but here are some questions you could reflect on in relation to the work you are doing for the throat chakra:

- To what degree do I experience the ability to express and communicate my sincere thoughts and feelings clearly and transparently?

- Do I dare to take space in the world? Do I make sure that I am visible and that my voice is heard?

- Do I know how to restrain my expression when needed, and sometimes to keep quiet?

- Am I able to listen to others' opinions and feelings?

- How do I cope with the sense of injustice?

- How capable do I feel of lecturing or writing in a way that can influence others? What could enhance this capacity?

- What is my relationship with creativity? Do I feel creative? What are the conditions for the flowering of my creative outlet?

Conclude the Day

This has been your encounter with the fifth dimension of your being, the dimension of expression represented by your throat chakra.

Express gratitude to this day. Recall what you have done throughout the day, either in terms of practice or intention. Recall events that may have been directly or indirectly associated with the learning of the chakra. Do not attempt to critically evaluate how much you have accomplished today. Even small steps are actual steps that you have taken, and you have certainly managed to stir not only this particular chakra but your entire chakra column toward a greater enlightenment.

Just before you go to sleep, prior to getting into bed or while already lying in it, bring your awareness to your throat chakra, behind your Adam's apple. Visualize that this chakra is superbly active, pulsating and rotating like a wheel that is spinning around its axis, thanks to your devoted attention today. Imagine that at the center of the wheel, there is a concentrated and highly potent point that is glowing with blue light.

Feel how this concentrated point of blue light begins to spread throughout the body, covering your legs all the way to your feet and extending to the top of your head. Feel how through this visualization, the chakra is releasing its unique consciousness and wisdom into both body and mind. Allow the chakra energy to reach any physical, emotional, or mental blocked area with its healing powers and to unravel and soothe it through its glowing blue light. Now your being as a whole, from head to toe, is radiating with blue light; even the surface of your skin is emitting this light.

Encompassed by this blue light, contemplate the greatest lesson of the throat chakra for a moment: You are able to experience an unconditional and independent sense of authenticity and clarity of being deep inside you, regardless of reactions, criticisms, or even injustices.

Now let the blue light dissolve back into the concentrated blue point. By dedicating your full attention to one chakra, you are now naturally and effortlessly taking a leap to the next one on the chakra ladder. For a brief moment, feel anticipation for tomorrow's frequency: the third eye chakra's Day of Wisdom.

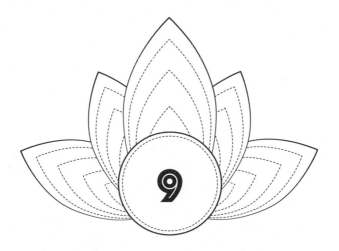

SATURDAY: ENGAGING THE THIRD EYE CHAKRA ON THE DAY OF WISDOM

Ajna chakra, known as the third eye, is most commonly depicted as a psychic eye located midway between the two physical eyes. Directly behind the eyebrow center, its gaze is turned inward rather than outward. Some systems argue that our chakra journey should commence from Ajna; being the seat of your inner guru, it commands all other chakras through its knowing, intuition, and understanding.[41] Saturday invites you to broaden your mind and turn it into a guiding source of clarity and insight.

---

41 Satyananda, *Kundalini Tantra*, 127–30.

Feel the Day of Wisdom

Good morning. You have just woken up to a day filled with the excitement of an extraordinary adventure: the opportunity to travel deep in the vast expanses of the intellectual realms. Equip yourself with nothing but curiosity and, if possible, bring your inner philosopher with you.

The chakras advise that a week should not pass without learning something new. The swift currents of worldly affairs can easily keep people busy with only the superficial layers of life, thus limiting the mind's capacities. Use the weekend's natural withdrawal from mundane commitments to take this shift inward. Make sure that your inner world does not remain dull and shallow.

Some erroneously think that the mind is a useless machine that takes us away from our heart, intuition, or spiritual nature. This is perhaps true if your mind is malnourished and heavily loaded with toxic mental chatter. If you misuse your mind by overthinking nonsense, you will end up believing that it is an uncreative element that leads to nothing besides more confusion and obscurity. If you feed your mind properly, you will soon realize that it rewards you with the elevating sense of supreme intelligence. Just as your body requires healthy nutrition and your heart requires emotional satisfaction, so too the mind gets hungry, and its ideal nourishment is letting in new thoughts, eye-opening ideas, and stimulating insights. Yes, this is definitely the day to dust off that book you've been meaning to read; maybe it's time to strain your brain to grasp Stephen Hawking's black hole theory!

Your incredible capacity as a human being is to pause and reflect from time to time. Make sense of your experience, raise deep questions, and wish to understand the "why" and the "how" of the world you live in. Saturday is your chance to consciously make yourself available to the enrichment of great thinkers and wise people while striving as much as possible to actively engage your own mind. Remember, the sixth chakra is all about *your* inner guru and the wisdom and perception that await deep within yourself.

While soaring to philosophical heights, you can use this bird's-eye view to widen your outlook on your life's journey. You yourself are an interesting study! Think about your life's themes and your main challenges and ponder where it is all leading. Whereas your Monday is a broad view of the structures and different aspects of your life, your Saturday allows you to observe the different pieces of the puzzle and to combine them into a new, enlightening way.

Recognize the Blessings

As you begin your day, open up to receive its radiant wisdom, gifts, and powers. Saturday's first grace lies in its capacity to expose you to the wisdom of the ages, whether philosophical, scientific, or spiritual. There are numerous wise ones who have blessed humanity with their profound perceptions. Their natural bend toward higher thinking can quickly awaken any sleepy mind. When unstimulated, our mind becomes sluggish, whereas proper inspiration encourages the mind to make a conscious effort to understand, including things that are not readily graspable.

A well-fed mind is not only intellectually satisfied but also more creative and efficient. That is why Sharma included a stage of learning in his well-known 5:00 a.m. daily practice. Claiming that the world belongs to learners, Sharma promotes the idea that increasing your rate of learning can make you far more success-ful.[42] By permitting new invigorating thoughts to enter and consciously directing your mind, you begin to replace the unnecessary, automatic thinking with informed and beneficial thoughts.

When the mind has no direction, it begins to roam and becomes foggy. This is where confusion creeps in. But with your intelligent element awake, you take back the mind's reins and bring the light of understanding into your life. The sixth chakra has been traditionally known as the monitoring center; its wide-open eye can bring order to your otherwise messy and conflicted emotions and feelings. It discards false thoughts with its sharp power of discrimination.

If you are open to receiving higher forms of wisdom, you will soon enjoy yet another of today's gifts: the ability to see your life in a more impersonal and universal context. To function at their best, third eyes must gain broad perspectives. We spend so much time laser-focused on the vast jigsaw puzzle of our life. When your third eye is open, however, it sees more parts of the picture; in this way, it can tell you what is meaningful and what is insignificant in your life. This is why you soar so high today: the higher you reach, the wiser you return to deal with your daily trivialities and challenges.

Use this day of wisdom to curiously discover unfamiliar areas of knowledge. Such excursions will help you realize that you are not only a passive learner; blending your mind with the great minds of others arouses your own philosophies and exciting thoughts. You will come to recognize that a hidden thinker exists in you, perhaps not as innovative as Socrates or da Vinci, but still enough to start trusting your intelligence and power of judgment.

---

42   Sharma, *5 AM Club*, 203.

And who knows, if you follow the trail marked by this day, it may even reveal psychic intuition and vision to your inner eye. The sixth chakra is, after all, the eye of the oracle, the element that sees into invisible realms of the universe and of yourself.

Connect with the Day's Happiness

Do you remember your early years when you were walking around with eager eyes, asking adults "Why?" and "How?" all day long? You have not lost this little philosopher in you, even if it has been momentarily buried beneath the thick layers of life's more immediate requirements and the belief that such questions are redundant or simply unanswerable. Today you have the chance to regain the ecstatic wish to know, this childlike curiosity in the face of a world full of magic.

There is, of course, the accompanying bliss of insight, when the universe generously grants you true knowledge. Think of Archimedes, the ancient Greek mathematician and inventor, who allegedly leapt out of his bathtub and ran naked through the streets of Syracuse, proclaiming *"Heurēka!"* ("I have found it!") after the sudden discovery of a natural law.[43] Thrilling discoveries are everywhere—even in your bathtub—if you only set your mind to it. Let your hidden questions resurface and lead you on your way to new realizations.

Saturday's happiness is all about the feeling that there is so much to learn. The world is exploding with mind-blowing ideas. Nowadays, they are one click away. Many people tend to over-specialize, narrowing their attention to only those things that directly affect their expertise and life management. Soon you

---

43 Toomer, "Archimedes."

end up thinking that you already know all that there is to know! Enjoy expanding your horizons and being lost in unexpected findings. Realize that the more you open to receive, the more you attract knowledge that can challenge your familiar frontiers. At the beginning of your week, you explored Tuesday's type of adventure: the adventure of intense experiences of body and feeling. Saturday is an adventure, but this is one that you undertake through your mind.

One more aspect of today's bliss is having your mind wide awake and positively alert. There is a great sense of health involved in the feeling of mental wakefulness, one that is not very different from the joy of a highly energetic body. The most basic nature of your mind is awareness; if you activate this sixth sense, you will realize that you have never been so alive and present.

Repeat These Affirmations

"Today ...

... I am life's excited student."

... I wish to be taught by humanity's greatest teachers."

... I open myself to life's riddles and mysteries."

... I am learning how to ask the right questions."

... I am attracting the knowledge that my mind is thirsty for."

... I am allowing my curiosity to show me the way."

... I am contacting the philosopher in me."

... I am entering the inner worlds of my deepest wisdom."

... I am learning to trust my intelligence and wisdom."

... I leap from trivial thoughts to the vast expanses of my mind."

Engage Your Third Eye Chakra

Learn something new. Decide that today you are going to find out something you do not know yet. This could be an expansion of the fields you are invested in; however, you can make it more stimulating by exposing yourself to fields that are not your cup of tea. Sometimes better insights come from unexpected encounters with very distant pathways of thought and knowledge.

Try to read or watch something that strains your brain. While cognitive science tells us that our brain's default is "cognitive ease"—avoiding any extra effort as long as things are going well—deliberate moments of "cognitive strain" can train your mind to stretch its capacities.[44] Concentrating only at work, when you must, will not do the trick. Be inspired by Wednesday's self-overcoming and think of today as a mental gym where you challenge yourself with less digestible ideas.

Choose any learning platform available to you. If you are unable to leave your house or workplace, read complex books or watch thoughtful lectures on YouTube. There are many hidden gems scattered online, including rare interviews and talks of twentieth-century giant thinkers. If possible, go to an eye-opening lecture or even to a one-day seminar.

Consider undertaking a new program of study. What system of knowledge or area of expertise would you, as life's student, immerse in? Enjoy the exhilarating experience of searching for such a long-term program. You never know when this acquired skill might suddenly become useful for you or for others.

Turn your current situation into a question that interests you. Even emotional states, such as heartbrokenness or jealousy, can be employed to ponder some essential questions about human

---

44   Kahneman, *Thinking, Fast and Slow*, 59–60.

life, the way our psyche works, and the nature of the world we live in. For instance, consider contemplating: "Is it possible to be completely free from emotional attachment?" Questions like that help you rise above your current state and realize that your situation is part of a universal condition. At times, universal perspectives may liberate you even more than an emotional release. If you are not occupied with any personal issue today, you can hold other questions within your mind, including those you haven't asked because they seem so utterly unattainable, such as "What is the meaning of life?" Aspire to gain at least one insight from your question by the end of the day.

Engage with friends in philosophical talks or spiritual inquiries. Instead of gossip and mundane chats, find time to sit together and raise bigger questions that you would like to clarify and explore together. Sometimes beautiful moments of intimacy take place between people who transcend trivialities to gain a shared insight. If you have no pressing questions, you can be aided by some philosophical, scientific, or spiritual text.

Target your confused or disturbing thoughts. Aside from arousing your higher mental capacities, use your Saturday to clear away unnecessary and self-destructive thinking. Are there any thoughts that visit you repeatedly and drain your being? Often we do not take the time to confront these mental shadows. Once identified, seek out an effective method that can uproot them from your mind, such as *The Work of Byron Katie*. In the same way, strive to make sense of emotions and feelings that you have not had the time to look into. This can be achieved through dialogue with a clear-minded friend, visiting a therapist, or reading a self-help book.

Practices to Empower Your Day

Activation. Smile into your third eye or use the chakra flowering meditation in chapter 3 to broadly open it up like a flower toward the world. Then rest your attention on the inner eye, behind the two physical eyes, as if you are looking at the world from this eye alone. This practice, which is presented in detail as this chapter's recommended daily meditation, activates the sixth chakra's inner knowing and vision. In general, try practicing looking at the world from the third eye throughout your entire Saturday, watching the world, people, and situations from this viewpoint alone.

Inspiration. Watch or read materials about any field of knowledge, from history to cosmology, the latest scientific research and discoveries, spiritual knowledge, philosophical ideas throughout human history, philosophers who expressed thought-provoking ideas, types of intelligence, improved ways of thinking, the capacities of the mind, the brain, the human psyche, questions you are passionate about, and so on.

Vision. Consider all the questions that arouse your curiosity. What are your questions at the moment? Visualize yourself fully opening up to depths of knowledge and wisdom, immersing yourself in higher thinking. What does it look like? Are there thoughts or other hindrances that limit your clarity and understanding? Decide on one thing that you are going to learn today and one practice to improve your thinking.

Recommended Meditation Practice

The third eye is a major contribution of ancient Indian thought; it is the understanding that between the two eyes, there is a third eye which ordinarily remains dormant. The third eye is the light of consciousness. Our two eyes cannot be used for inward perception and realization because they can only look outwardly; they have to be closed. We are able to turn our gaze inward using the third eye. The easiest way to stimulate this dormant eye is by closing your eyes and then focusing on the space in between the two eyebrows. This is one of the simplest methods of being attentive.

The third eye is a magnet for attention. If you give attention to it, your attention becomes magnetically drawn to it and absorbed in it. Something extraordinary takes place when you are fixing your attention there—the third eye concentrates all your mind energy. With this simple focus, your mental energy can no longer be wasted. Thoughts are moving in front of you, passing like clouds in the sky, but you are unable to identify with them. Centering yourself in the third eye is not like centering yourself in your thoughts; the third eye is more like the free and silent observer of thoughts.

• • • • •

Place your palms on your closed eyes for at least five minutes. Allow your palms to touch the eyeballs, but do so with little pressure, like a feather resting on your eyes. Use less and less pressure until you are touching as if not touching, as if your hands have no weight. When you slightly touch the eyeballs with your palms, subtle energy begins to move within. You will be able to feel lightness spreading all over your face and head, making you buoyant from within.

Slowly, the energy falling back from the eyes will hit the third eye, and perhaps from the third eye it will also drip into your heart. Allow your heart to open to receive this downward flow from the third eye. When your eyes are silent and relaxed and the energy is moving from them to the third eye, thoughts will naturally stop.

Remove your palms from your eyes and, with your eyes still closed, let your two eyes center on the middle of your forehead, feeling the point of the third eye. When you have reached the point, your eyes will become fixed. Notice how the third eye concentrates all your mind's energy and how you become pure awareness, separate from thoughts. After at least fifteen minutes of focusing on your third eye, slowly and gently open your eyes.

Today, look at the world—both the inner world and the outer world—from your third eye. Imagine that you have only one eye and that your two physical eyes are secondary. What does the world look like? What do your thoughts look like? Close your eyes whenever possible and—even if only for a moment—place yourself at the deeper point, not only between the eyes but also behind the eyes. Pay attention to how your mind is easily silenced in this way; realize that you are coming into contact with yourself as pure awareness.

Other Practices

- Add purple—the third eye chakra's color of depth and original thinking—to your clothes, workplace, or home.

- Consume foods and superfoods that feed your brain. Blueberries, broccoli, nuts, seeds, dark chocolate, avocados, and whole grains are all well-researched examples.

- Sharpen your brain with games like riddles, quizzes, and puzzles. There are also plenty of mental workouts out there. Try Neurobic exercises that introduce your brain to small new experiences, such as brushing your teeth with your nondominant hand or switching around your morning activities.

- Develop a creative idea. Choose any vision that exists in a potential state inside you—such as a vague concept of a novel you have always wished to write—and strive to expand, elucidate, and structure it as much as possible. Transforming an elusive thought into a clear, well-explained idea is an excellent practice for your third eye.

- Become your own teacher. You can do that by allowing your deepest thoughts to pour out on paper. Give voice to insight, slowly realizing that there is wisdom in you. One way to trigger this is by asking yourself important questions. Close your eyes and visualize a manifestation of yourself in your wisest, most mature form. Ask a question and let your inner guru respond. Even if you do not understand the answer, write it down. You can share the answers with others and discuss their meaning and implications.

- Tell and retell your life narrative. As the narrator of the story of your life, you hold the power to reshape it in a liberating and enhancing way. Look for techniques and books that help reset any unconscious storytelling. Construct a story full of possibilities and growth opportunities.

- Learn to master and own your mind. Any meditations that develop concentration or neutral observation of thoughts and feelings can be helpful. Jack Kornfield's meditation, A Mind Like Sky, can help you develop a mind that is vast like space, where thoughts can appear and disappear without conflict.

- Discover the sixth chakra as a gateway to inner journeys and dimensions. You can achieve this by experimenting with third-eye practices that develop psychic vision and intuition.[45] Lucid dreaming and channeling are examples of such an activation.

• Try Shri Yantra meditation. Yantras are ancient geometrical designs based on the principles of sacred geometry; Shri Yantra is considered the queen of yantras. Gazing into Shri Yantra is a profound third-eye meditation that enables your consciousness to go beyond the normal framework of the mind.

• Engage your mind in spiritual self-inquiry. Spiritual masters, such as the twentieth-century mystic Ramana Maharshi, have recommended using questions to attain inner illumination. Maharshi's particular question was "Who am I?", a form of investigation into the nature of the mind. In Zen Buddhism, Koans are employed for the same purpose. Koans are mind-boggling riddles used by Zen masters to evoke nonverbal understanding in their students. There are also scriptures that provoke self-inquiry, such as the centuries-old Hindu text *Yoga Vasistha*.

Notice the Challenges

Be aware whether it is time to face certain issues that arise from your Saturday encounter with the intellectual center of your being.

Detect possible mental laziness, even while reading about the sixth chakra challenge. Pay attention to whether your mind is too foggy, confused, and overloaded to participate in the Day of Wisdom. Do you identify yourself as an emotional or physical person who cannot possibly be interested in developing intellect? Look for any resistance you might have to new ideas. Do you have a

---

45   Satyananada, *Kundalini Tantra*, 129, 214–18.

feeling that you already know too much? Notice a possible mistrust you may have of your own intelligence and wisdom. Do you believe that you are incapable of mental brightness? Examine whether you were conditioned to think about studying a certain way; it could be due to school trauma or disappointing experiences related to learning from authority.

You can either contemplate these challenges in writing or look for methods of teaching that guide you on your way to resolving them.

Journal

Have a journal or a notebook on hand to record your thoughts and observations throughout the day. Feel free to take any direction in your writing, but here are some questions you could reflect on in relation to the work you are doing for the third eye chakra:

- To what degree do I experience an awake, passionate, fresh, and curious mind?
- Do I feel thirsty for knowledge?
- Do I have room for new dimensions of exploration and learning?
- Do I enjoy expanding my understanding about the world and about myself?
- Do I know how to engage in philosophical thoughts? Do I know how to pose questions and inquire into them?
- Can I find the inner guru that responds to my innermost questions?
- Am I capable of receiving and absorbing words of wisdom?

• Can I listen to my own thoughts and discern which are constructive and which are irrelevant to my growth and development?

Conclude the Day

This has been your encounter with the sixth dimension of your being, the dimension of wisdom represented by your third eye chakra.

Express gratitude to this day. Recall what you have done throughout the day, either in terms of practice or intention. Recall events that may have been directly or indirectly associated with the learning of the chakra. Do not attempt to critically evaluate how much you have accomplished today. Even small steps are actual steps that you have taken, and you have certainly managed to stir not only this particular chakra but your entire chakra column toward a greater enlightenment.

Just before you go to sleep, prior to getting into bed or while already lying in it, bring your awareness to your third eye chakra, behind the brow. Visualize that this chakra is superbly active, pulsating and rotating like a wheel that is spinning around its axis, thanks to your devoted attention throughout this day. Imagine that at the center of the wheel, there is a concentrated and highly potent point that is glowing with purple light.

Feel how this concentrated point of purple light begins to spread throughout the body, covering your legs all the way to your feet and extending to the top of your head. Feel how through this visualization, the chakra is releasing its unique consciousness and wisdom into both body and mind. Allow the chakra energy to reach any physical, emotional, or mental blocked area with its healing powers and to unravel and soothe it through its glowing purple light. Now your being as a whole, from head to toe, is radiating with purple light; even the surface of your skin is emitting this light.

Encompassed by this purple light, contemplate the greatest lesson of the third eye chakra for a moment: You are able to experience an unconditional and independent mind deep inside you that is lucid, awake, and wise; it remains unaffected even by noisy, turbulent, and constantly changing thoughts.

Now let the purple light dissolve back into the concentrated purple point. By dedicating your full attention to one chakra, you are now naturally and effortlessly taking a leap to the next one on the chakra ladder. For a brief moment, feel anticipation for tomorrow's frequency: the crown chakra's Day of Spirit.

SUNDAY: ENGAGING THE CROWN CHAKRA ON THE DAY OF SPIRIT

At the highest point of your being, the center of your skullcap, the crown chakra (Sahasrara) resides. Some say it is not a chakra at all, but the culmination of the progressive ascension through the chakras.[46] This is the center of transcendence, where you are elevated beyond time and space, mundane awareness, and the world as you know it. It is like sitting on the vertex of a mountaintop, from which your life seems like a miniature landscape. Sunday gives you permission to travel that high and to leave the concerns of all other chakras behind.

---

46 Satyananda, *Kundalini Tantra*, 189.

Feel the Day of Spirit

Good morning. You have just woken up to a day of complete restfulness, where time stops and deep silence permeates your home and your being. Remind yourself of the biblical story of creation—if God could feel content after a long week of creation and retire from all action, why shouldn't you? Today, allow total abandonment of the constant rush forward.

It is a time to rest your mind and heart by feeling that you can inwardly let go and be deeply untroubled. At least today, the world can manage without you. You are finally free to turn your full attention to your innermost being. Luckily, Sunday's increased collective quietude endorses your choice to make this shift and remain guilt-free.

During the week you were focused on the active, changing, progressing aspect of the world and of yourself. Now it is time to honor the other half: the still, unchanging part of your being. This part is always there, sharing the eternal ground of all creation. You do not need to make an effort to reach it. It is more like tuning in to the right radio station, the one that only plays silence as the background music of the world. The seventh day is your chance to listen to this music and to participate in creation's seventh day: the meditation of the universe.

Today is for timelessness. Forget that prior to Sunday there was a week at all. Give no thought to the day after or to the week that follows. It is a little bit like Tuesday, which celebrates life in the here and now, yet Sunday goes much deeper. Consider it a non-day between the weeks, an island surrounded by a sea of peace.

If you faithfully follow this day's potential, it will profoundly replenish your being, uprooting and clearing away any tensions or pressures accumulated in your body and mind. If you do it right, it will lead you to a new cycle of creation, glowing and light. This requires some trust on your part that you can fully withhold all work commitments as well as any thoughts or worries about your life's unresolved issues. Soon, trust will be replaced by the understanding that such a suspension is also a better strategy. If you rejuvenate in the deepest sense, you will actually return to your daily life more insightful and capable of unraveling those issues.

Recognize the Blessings

As you begin your day, open up to receive its radiant wisdom, gifts, and powers. The crown chakra is a part of ourselves that is rarely acknowledged because, in so many ways, it does not constitute a vital part of human life. While some feel called to attain profound spiritual states as their ultimate and noblest destination, you do not have to be among them to benefit from the unique perspective of this chakra. Dedicating just one day a week will illuminate this unknown layer of your being and fulfill its crucial role in this integrative path. After you have given your heart, mind, and body to life's six active aspects, the seventh chakra day is the one missing lesson that can make your life complete.

What today's teaching holds for you is the reminder that, beyond life's ever-changing conditions and your own fluctuating moods, thoughts, and emotions, there is an unchanging, utterly independent being in you that has remained unaffected since the beginning of time. It is like outer space, which contains countless stars, or the vast blue sky that accommodates passing clouds while remaining utterly uninfluenced. This is what the seventh day strives to point at: the indestructible element that hides behind all your social and personality identities.

Today you will learn the importance of coming into contact with this innermost part because as soon as it awakens, it releases you from attachment, fear, dependency, and lack. This inner being does not require the world to be complete and content; thus, it allows you to be happy instead of waiting for external events to bring you happiness. From this profound perspective, you do not really "need" that other person to love you, nor do you "have" to be promoted at work to achieve satisfaction. Happiness becomes an internal matter, a quality of being that is completely in your own hands.

If you merge your being with this day's blessings, it will reveal to you an authentic inner stability where nothing can change your world. Such stability will quickly and efficiently quiet the week's turmoil, absorbing overdoing as well as overthinking in its silence. At the same time, by becoming familiar with this part of you that cannot suffer, you will be able to move on to another week cycle less dependent and, therefore, less fearful and anxious. You will become capable of commanding your mind from a nonattached, otherworldly point of view.

The secret is that activity cannot be complete or balanced without its opposite—nonactivity—in the same way that sound cannot exist without silence. You need this other part of yourself to liberate your action from tension. When you know that you exist even without doing and that you can be happy even without fulfilling any of your future plans, your action in the world becomes freer. For this to be established, initiate contact with the unexplored expanses of your innermost being today.

Connect with the Day's Happiness

The Hindu ashrama system believes that any individual should follow four age-based life stages. From the age of forty-eight onward (after the individual has faithfully completed the student and household phases), one is encouraged to detach from the world and to immerse in spiritual affairs; this is called the retired phase, which is followed by the renunciation phase.[47] Contemplate the feeling of final release from worldly engagement, a moment when you can allow yourself to soar freely in the open skies of your spirit.

For the most part, people are deeply occupied and troubled, helplessly trying to accommodate all that life brings up during the week. We easily forget our core. That is why today's happiness is, before anything else, the joy of being unconcerned. It is just like traveling to a faraway destination, somewhere the political news of the world cannot reach—so long as you are there, nothing happens in the world except for sunsets and the murmur of the sea. The world's problems exist only through your awareness of them. Today, be blissfully unaware, even of your own troubles.

Taking this healthy distance, you can also tap into the happiness of being alone. No one can be complete without relationships and fulfilling interactions, and Tuesdays and Thursdays ensure that you do not forget this message. But today you can afford to feel the fullness of being with yourself, devoted to self-exploration, without the need to relate or to be someone for somebody.

Paradoxically, in such a deep solitude, you can open up to the greatest bliss of the crown chakra: the loss of your individual boundaries, which makes it possible for you to realize your inseparability from the universal spirit. It is crucial to have a

---

47   Nugteren, *Belief, Bounty, and Beauty*, 13–21.

well-targeted and determined self, and to that you devote your Wednesdays and Fridays. Yet, at the end of the day, you ought to remember that your body and mind belong to a greater whole. You do not need to carry the entire weight of this life on your shoulders; you share it with the unfathomable mystery from which this life has sprung.

Repeat These Affirmations

"Today …

… I allow myself to leave the world behind."

… I have nothing to do and nowhere to go."

… I am allowing timelessness to take over."

… I am immersing my mind and heart in the silence of my innermost being."

… I am relaxing and tuning in to the meditation of the universe."

… I am realizing that the background music of the world is silence."

… I am falling into the gap between my thoughts."

… I am getting in touch with the eternal in me."

… I am delving into the vast expanses of my being."

Engage Your Crown Chakra

As much as possible, put aside your smartphone and laptop and keep away from the news and your television. You may even hide your clock or watch to foster the sense of timelessness.

Make time to be with yourself in solitude. Observing complete silence for several hours, or even taking a full day of silence, is particularly powerful. Feel how, through the practice of refraining from speech, you place yourself in an unworldly position.

Go for long walks and simply be while contemplating the miracle of creation or feeling free from your worldly identity. Spending quiet time in nature can be ideal, since nature easily echoes the meditation of the universe.

Be a yogi for a day and sit for long meditations. Enjoy steeping your being in the state of open and unfocused awareness. When meditation is not a part of the day but the very fragrance of the day, you may find it far easier to relax your mind and body into silent sitting.

While engaged in mundane activities, notice that every action takes place against the backdrop of nonaction and stillness. Be aware of the immovable axis that all activities happen around.

Read scriptures—such as the Old or New Testament, the Hindu Vedas and Upanishads, the Buddhist Heart Sutra, or the Quran—to get in touch with the ancient wisdom of the world's religions.

Attend spiritual gatherings. These can be teachings, group meditations, or circles of sacred music or mantras. You can also invite your friends to meditate with you; a collective sharing of the day's energy field could deepen and enhance it.

Watch videos or listen to audio recordings of spiritual teachers and thinkers. Contemplate eternal truths and questions by yourself, such as "Who am I?" Another option is to take a short or ongoing course on meditation, inner peace, or the still mind.

Identify your worldly attachments and see if you can let them go, even a little. What keeps you tied to the earth, making you unable to "disappear" for a day?

Create a sacred atmosphere at home using incense, meditative music, candles, and images of meditating figures. For a day, make your space temple-like. Remember that Saturday and Sunday have been considered occasions for the elevation of spirit. Preserve this sense of specialness, even if you do not attend church, synagogue, or mosque.

Keep your body light and unburdened to support the day's element of air. This can be accomplished through fresh eating—mainly raw foods, vegetables and fruits, and juices—or a day of water fasting. Juice fasting, the abstinence from all food and drink except for water and fresh vegetable juices, is a popular variation. Chemist and nutrition expert Raymond Francis recommends making a habit of fasting one day a week to promote detoxification and, ultimately, to extend the life span.[48] Of course, if you have certain medical conditions, consult your doctor prior to fasting. Another way to remove stored toxins is by using hyperthermic (sweat) treatments, such as a dry sauna.

Practices to Empower Your Day

Activation. Smile into your crown chakra or use the chakra flowering meditation in chapter 3 to open it up like a flower toward the heavens, feeling the opening of the crown as if it were connected by a thread to the infinite space above your head. You can also start by listening to some sacred, spiritual, or celestial music. Another simple way to initiate your day is by immediately shifting from your lying down position to sitting and meditating on your bed—just like Sri Yukteswar, the guru of the renowned twentieth-century Indian yogi Yogananda, who would, after "abrupt halt of stupendous snores, a sigh or two, and perhaps a bodily movement," move at once to a sitting position and enter a state of "deep yogic joy."[49]

---

48   Francis, *Never Feel Old Again*, 194–98.

49   Yogananda, *Autobiography of a Yogi*, 106.

Inspiration. Watch or read materials about spiritual enlighten-ment, scriptures, spiritual guidance, Satsang (a traditional spir-itual dialogue with an enlightened master), spiritual music and mantras, meditation, monasteries, the mystery of existence, the nature of consciousness, the meaning of death, the end of suf-fering, spiritual traditions, spiritual masters and saints, Kund-alini and the subtle body, and so on.

Vision. Consider how you could connect more deeply to silence and notice the unchanging during your Sunday. Visualize yourself in a Zen state today—what does it look like? Are there blockages that keep you from fully sinking into silence and freedom from the world? Finally, decide on one activity and one practice that will carry you deeper into your inner stillness.

Recommended Meditation Practice

This gentle process, called the golden light meditation, originated with Osho.[50] It imitates a natural energetic process that takes place in your subtle body when it is awake and active. Golden light is penetrating your body through the top of your head all the way down, while your life force responds to it by flowing all the way up to the top of the head. The penetrating light is the masculine energy to which feminine energy responds. Together they form a beautiful circle, a subtle love affair. Since this flow is like subtle inhalation and exhalation, synchronize this visualiza-tion with the inhale and the exhale.

• • • • •

---

50   Osho, *Meditation*, 133–35.

You can either lie down on your back or sit on your meditation chair. Close your eyes. When you breathe in, visualize golden light entering your head and spreading through your body, as if the sun has risen close to your head. The golden light is pouring into your head, moving deeply inside you and through you, until it pours out through your toes. Use this visualization for each inhalation. When you breathe out, visualize darkness entering through your toes, a great dark river that rises and exits through the head. Use this visualization for each exhalation.

As the golden light enters, let it cleanse your whole body. Think of it like a masculine energy that cleanses and fills you with creative force. And as the darkness comes from your toes, visualize it as the darkest color you can conceive flowing through you in a river-like movement. This is a feminine energy; this dark energy can soothe your body and mind and make you more receptive, calm, and restful.

Make your breathing slow and deep so you can visualize fully. Go as slowly as possible with a deeply rested body. Continue these visualizations for at least fifteen minutes.

After you finish meditating, while you are engaged in daily activities, visualize in sync with your inhalations and exhalations whenever you remember to. Even visualizing just one of the movements, either the golden light or the dark river, can be effective. Feel how this visualization immediately links you to the world beyond—a subtle world in which these visions are an invisible but tangible reality.

This meditation could also be a beautiful way to close your Sunday. Lie down in your bed, relax, and—when you feel that you are half asleep—visualize golden light and the dark river for up to twenty minutes. The darkness around you echoes the dark river that flows through you with every exhale. This practice will then flow into your unconscious once you have fallen asleep.

Other Practices

- Meditate on all seven chakras to experience them as one. Obviously Sunday is governed by the crown chakra, but bear in mind that this chakra gathers the other six into one column of whole-body awakening. A good metaphor for this is a prism that breaks white light into seven colors that then return, in the opposite direction, to become pure light once again. You can visualize precisely that! Imagine how the central column that pierces through the center of your body reabsorbs all the seven rainbow layers that emanated from your inner being during the week, transforming them into one glowing, golden-white thread. In the same way, you can also practice full chakra awakening, such as smiling into your chakras or the chakra flowering meditation, both found in chapter 3.

- Do slow yoga asanas (postures) and gentle breathing exercises like Nadi Shodhana. In slow yoga, you rest longer in each posture to enter a meditative state of mind-body unity. Nadi Shodhana is alternate nostril breathing that enables you to equalize the air moving in and out of your nostrils, thus promoting peace of mind. One more significant yogic practice you can experiment with is the Kriya Yoga set of practices.[51]

- Meditate on the gap between your thoughts. By shifting your attention to the gap between thoughts rather than the thoughts themselves, you are moving from the world of objects to the world of space and consciousness. Realize just how much space there is between thoughts. In this

---

51   Satyananda, *Kundalini Tantra*, 284–315.

way, you will find that your mind is a vast expanse that contains thoughts, but it is not made of thoughts.

• Spend an hour in a dark room. Dark-room meditation is a highly effective way to swiftly reveal timelessness and inner space. Various spiritual traditions have employed dark-room techniques as a way of obtaining deep spiritual growth. In today's day and age, we have lost touch with complete darkness. It is quite easy to create your own dark room experience at home: in any way possible, prevent even the slightest stream of light into a room. Then sit or lie down, either in complete silence or with some soft music in the background.

• Try Zazen. The ultimate Zen Buddhist practice focuses on a particular posture that unifies body and mind. Zazen is sitting itself. If you are well-positioned, immersion in the here and now takes place by itself.

• Other traditional Sunday practices can include the variety of death meditations. There are Buddhist meditations, for example, that involve visualizing the decay of your own body or contemplating the inevitability of your own death.

• Any practice that involves the awakening of the central column—the main subtle nerve channel that pierces through the center of the body—can be highly suitable for the Day of Spirit. Activating the central channel is the key to spiritual transcendence. It enables an anti-gravitational flow of your life force toward the highest point of your being, which is the crown chakra. Try the Tibetan vase-breathing meditation or the Taoist microcosmic orbit meditation.[52]

---

52   See Yeshe, *Bliss of Inner Fire* and Chia, *Awaken Healing Energy.*

Notice the Challenges

Be aware whether it is time to face certain issues that arise from your Sunday encounter with the spiritual center of your being.

Observe whether you find it hard to remain in silence—is your mind noisier than ever or seeking distractions? Examine whether this day of non-doing is a challenge for your addiction to action and for your identity as a doer. Be watchful if your thoughts are occupied with unresolved issues, driven by the wish to remain in control at all times. Look into any struggles you may have with being alone. When you are in solitude, do you feel lonely rather than content? Take notice of fears you may be confronted with, such as the fear of death or the fear of losing ground, when entering deep meditation. Identify untreated issues in your relationship with "God" or spirit. Do you hold on to the belief that you are an outcast of the divine reality? Pay attention to whether you feel too physically heavy to enjoy Sunday's atmosphere of lightness and transparency.

You can either contemplate these challenges in writing or look for methods of teaching that guide you on your way to resolving them.

Journal

Have a journal or a notebook on hand to record your thoughts and observations throughout the day. Feel free to take any direction in your writing, but here are some questions you could reflect on in relation to the work you are doing for the crown chakra:

- To what degree am I able to close my eyes and immerse in meditation?
- Do I find it possible to keep quiet?

- Do I easily make friends with myself when I am completely alone?

- Do I feel that it is possible for me to put worldly affairs aside for a day and enjoy timelessness?

- Do I experience attachment to certain activities, social roles, thoughts, or emotions that hinder my ability to rest inside myself?

- Do I feel capable of contacting the spiritual dimension of life?

- Can I identify in myself a deeper existence that has nothing to do with my external appearance?

- Do I trust that I possess an inherently enlightened nature?

Conclude the Day

This has been your encounter with the seventh dimension of your being, the dimension of spirit represented by your crown chakra.

Express gratitude to this day. Recall what you have done throughout the day, either in terms of practice or intention. Recall events that may have been directly or indirectly associated with the learning of the chakra. Do not attempt to critically evaluate how much you have accomplished today. Even small steps are actual steps that you have taken, and you have certainly managed to stir not only this particular chakra but your entire chakra column toward a greater enlightenment.

Just before you go to sleep, prior to getting into bed or while already lying in it, bring your awareness to your crown chakra, centered on the top of your head. Visualize that this chakra is superbly active, pulsating and rotating like a wheel that is spinning around its axis, thanks to your devoted attention throughout this day. Imagine that at the center of the wheel, there is a concentrated and highly potent point that is glowing with white light.

Feel how this concentrated point of white light begins to spread throughout the body, covering your legs all the way to your feet and extending to the top of your head. Feel how through this visualization, the chakra is releasing its unique consciousness and wisdom into both body and mind. Allow the chakra energy to reach any physical, emotional, or mental blocked area with its healing powers and to unravel and soothe it through its glowing white light. Now your being as a whole, from head to toe, is radiating with white light; even the surface of your skin is emitting this light.

Encompassed by this white light, contemplate the greatest lesson of the crown chakra for a moment: You are able to experience an innermost self deep inside you, one that remains forever unlimited, universal, and luminous, inaccessible to the effects of time and even death.

Now let the white light dissolve back into the concentrated white point. By dedicating your full attention to one chakra, you are now naturally and effortlessly taking a leap to the next one on the chakra ladder. For a brief moment, feel anticipation toward your next seven-day cycle and tomorrow's frequency: the root chakra Day of Grounding.

CONCLUSION

At this point, a complete way of life is laid out before you, all thanks to the ancient wisdom of the chakras.

Getting to know the chakras as a total practice, a roadmap for life itself, is radically different from learning about them theoretically and practicing them on occasion. Now you know the chakras as an easy and clear way to nourish and realize all the different parts of your being, a way of growing the various flowers in your life's garden.

What the chakras offer you is the power to create your life, to give shape to your life's experience through an inspiration that literally emerges from your innermost being. In the words of author and artist José Argüelles, the chakras show you how to replace the soul-draining equation "Time is money" with the equation "Time is art."[53] This might be a radical shift in the way you have been thinking about how individuals can lead their lives, manage their time, and fulfill their hidden potentials.

This change—and its many implications—cannot take place overnight. Start gently and pay attention to feedback, the way your

---

53   Argüelles, "Law of Time."

inner being responds, the inevitable ripples that spread to your environment. Even if you begin by fulfilling only one-tenth of all that is offered in this book, this should be more than enough for a significant leap in your self-development and self-leadership. Moreover, a little reorientation followed by some practice will already begin to pour a greater sense of meaning into your experience of daily life: the way you wake up in the morning knowing what expects you as soon as you open your eyes, the way you feel on the threshold of a new week, and the way you feel when you conclude a week and approach Sunday's big reset. Every morning you will rise to a new frequency; your week will feel rich and diverse, revealing one of its different facets each day, like a brilliant diamond.

It is my sincere wish that you will slowly become tuned in to this path, and that this will happen not because of self-discipline but because of initial steps and small experiments that will naturally draw your heart, mind, and body to a new flow. I hope that by following this rhythm of seven, you will be gratified with the taste of a holistic experience of life, and that this sense of all-embracing flowering will show you the way. Above all, my wish for you is that your wise chakras will endow you with a truly spiritual experience of your week that will take you beyond the repetitive cycle of work and rest, revealing farther and yet unknown horizons of your being.

BIBLIOGRAPHY

Ackerman, Courtney E. "What Is Self-Transcendence? Definition and 6 Examples (+PDF)." PositivePsychology. September 1, 2020. https://positivepsychology.com/self -transcendence/.

Argüelles, José. "The Law of Time." Foundation for the Law of Time. Accessed October 6, 2020. https://lawoftime.org /lawoftime.html.

Chia, Mantak. *Awaken Healing Energy through the Tao: The Taoist Secret of Circulating Internal Power*. Santa Fe, NM: Aurora Press, 1983.

———. *Healing Love through the Tao: Cultivating Female Sexual Energy*. Rochester, VT: Destiny Books, 2005.

Dalai Lama and Howard C. Cutler. "The Art of Happiness Quotes" from *The Art of Happiness: A Handbook for Living*. Goodreads. Accessed October 5, 2020. https://www .goodreads.com/work/quotes/1651617-the-art-of-happiness -a-handbook-for-living.

Easwaran, Eknath, trans. *The Upanishads*. 2nd ed. Tomales, CA: Nilgiri, 2007.

Eisler, Melissa. "Laughter Meditation: 5 Healing Benefits and a 10-Minute Practice." Chopra. March 10, 2017. https://chopra.com/articles/laughter-meditation-5-healing-benefits-and-a-10-minute-practice.

Fernando, Anushka B. P., Jennifer E. Murray, and Amy L. Milton. "The Amygdala: Securing Pleasure and Avoiding Pain." *Frontiers in Behavioral Neuroscience* 7 (December 2013). https://doi.org/10.3389/fnbeh.2013.00190.

Francis, Raymond. *Never Fear Cancer Again: How to Prevent and Reverse Cancer.* Deerfield Beach, FL: Health Communications, Inc., 2011.

———. *Never Feel Old Again: Aging Is a Mistake—Learn How to Avoid It.* Deerfield Beach, FL: Health Communications, Inc., 2013.

Frankl, Viktor E. *Man's Search for Meaning.* Boston: Beacon Press, 2006.

"Get Grounded and Thrive This Fall By Eating These 5 Foods." Simple Mills. September 26, 2018. https://simplemills.com/Learn/Blog/Blog-Posting/September-2018/Get-Grounded-and-Thrive-This-Fall-By-Eating-These.aspx.

Gurdjieff and the Fourth Way. "Self-Remembering." Learning Institute for Growth, Healing, and Transformation. http://www.gurdjiefffourthway.org/pdf/SELF-REMEMBERING.pdf.

Hallowell, A. Irving. "Temporal Orientation in Western Civilization and in a Pre-Literate Society." *American Anthropologist* 39, no. 4 (1937): 647–70. Accessed May 26, 2020. www.jstor.org/stable/662420.

Hedegaard, Erik. "Wim Hof Says He Holds the Key to a Healthy Life—But Will Anyone Listen?" *Rolling Stone*. November 3, 2017. https://www.rollingstone.com/culture/culture -features/wim-hof-says-he-holds-the-key-to-a-healthy -life-but-will-anyone listen-196647/.

Jeffrey, Scott. "Cultivate Boundless Energy with an Ancient Standing Meditation Called Zhan Zhuang." CEOsage. Accessed October 5, 2020. https://scottjeffrey.com/zhan -zhuang/.

Judith, Anodea. "History of the Chakra System." Sacred Centers. Accessed October 5, 2020. http://sacredcenters.com/history -of-the-chakra-system/.

Kabat-Zinn, Jon. "The Body Scan Meditation." Palouse Mindfulness. 2005. https://palousemindfulness.com/docs/bodyscan .pdf.

———. "Mountain Meditation Script." Palouse Mindfulness. Accessed October 5, 2020. https://palousemindfulness.com /docs/mountain meditation.pdf.

Kahneman, Daniel. *Thinking, Fast and Slow*. London: Penguin, 2012.

Kowalski, Kyle. "What Is Transcendence? The True Top of Maslow's Hierarchy of Needs." Sloww. Accessed October 5, 2020. https://www.sloww.co/transcendence-maslow/.

Li, Qing. "'Forest Bathing' Is Great for Your Health. Here's How to Do It." *Time*. May 1, 2018. https://time.com/5259602 /japanese-forest-bathing/.

McLeod, Saul. "Maslow's Hierarchy of Needs." SimplyPsychology. Updated March 20, 2020. http://www.simplypsychology .org/maslow.html.

Nhat Hanh, Thich. "Walk like a Buddha." *Tricycle*, Summer 2011. https://tricycle.org/magazine/walk-buddha/.

Nugteren, Albertina. *Belief, Bounty, and Beauty: Rituals Around Sacred Trees in India*. Leiden, Netherlands: Brill Academic Publishers, 2005.

Osho. *Meditation: The First and Last Freedom*. New York: St. Martin's Griffin, 2004.

Pandita, Sayadaw U. "What Is Vipassana Meditation and How Do You Practice It?" Lion's Roar. March 3, 2020. https://www.lionsroar.com/how-to-practice-vipassana-insight-meditation/.

Rana, Sarika. "Here's Why Eating Food with Hands Is a Healthy Habit." NDTV Food. Updated April 3, 2018. https://food.ndtv.com/health/heres-why-eating-food-with-hands-is-a-healthy-habit-1831872.

Riggio, Ronald E. "There's Magic in Your Smile." *Psychology Today*. June 25, 2012. https://www.psychologytoday.com/intl/blog/cutting-edge-leadership/201206/there-s-magic-in-your-smile.

Satyananda Saraswati, Swami. *Kundalini Tantra*. Munger, Bihar, India: Yoga Publications Trust, 2012.

Sharma, Robin. *The 5 AM Club: Own Your Morning. Elevate Your Life*. New York: HarperCollins, 2020.

Spiritual Awakening. "Om Mani Padme Hum, Most Powerful Third Eye Opening Meditation—Third Eye Activation." YouTube. December 28, 2017. https://www.youtube.com/watch?v=v0IRF4gUcc0&t=590s.

Thorp, Tris. "Guided Meditation: Ground Yourself Using the Earth Element." Chopra. February 4, 2019. https://chopra

.com/articles/guided-meditation-ground-yourself
-using-the-earth-element.

Toomer, Gerald J. "Archimedes." *Encyclopaedia Britannica Online*. Last modified November 12, 2019. https://www
.britannica.com/biography/Archimedes.

Traditional Music Channel. "African Zulu Drum Music." YouTube. March 7, 2014. https://www.youtube.com
/watch?v=BLZTOiKBHVA.

Tubali, Shai. *The Seven Chakra Personality Types: Discover the Energetic Forces That Shape Your Life, Your Relationships, and Your Place in the World*. Newburyport, MA: Conari Press, 2018.

———. *Unlocking the 7 Secret Powers of the Heart: A Practical Guide to Living in Trust and Love*. Rochester, VT: Earthdancer Books, 2018.

Wallis, Christopher. "The Real Story on the Chakras." Hareesh. February 5, 2016. https://hareesh.org/blog/2016/2/5/the
-real-story-on-the-chakras.

Wood, Wendy. *Good Habits, Bad Habits: The Science of Making Positive Changes That Stick*. New York: Farrar, Straus and Giroux, 2019.

Yogananda, Paramhansa. *Autobiography of a Yogi*. Los Angeles: Self-Realization Fellowship, 2011.

Zerubavel, Eviatar. *The Seven Day Circle: The History and Meaning of the Week*. Chicago: University of Chicago Press, 1985.

RECOMMENDED READING

Chapter 3: Chakra Personality Types and the Seven-Day Cycle

Chia, Mantak. *The Inner Smile: Increasing Chi through the Cultivation of Joy*. Rochester, VT: Destiny Books, 2008.

Chapter 4: Monday: Engaging the Root Chakra on the Day of Grounding

Jeffrey, Scott. "Cultivate Boundless Energy with an Ancient Standing Meditation Called Zhan Zhuang." CEOsage. Accessed October 5, 2020. https://scottjeffrey.com/zhan -zhuang/.

Kabat-Zinn, Jon. "The Body Scan Meditation." Palouse Mindfulness. 2005. https://palousemindfulness.com/docs/bodyscan .pdf.

Kissel Wegela, Karen. "How to Practice Mindfulness Meditation." *Psychology Today*. January 19, 2010. https://www .psychologytoday.com/us/blog/the-courage-be-present /201001/how-practice-mindfulness-meditation.

Moyer, Nancy. "14 Leg Massage Ideas." Healthline. July 17, 2019. https://www.healthline.com/health/leg-massage.

Nortje, Alicia. "How to Practice Mindfulness: 10 Practical Steps and Tips." PositivePsychology. September 1, 2020. https://positivepsychology.com/how-to-practice-mindfulness/.

Pandita, Sayadaw U. "What Is Vipassana Meditation and How Do You Practice It?" Lion's Roar. March 3, 2020. https://www.lionsroar.com/how-to-practice-vipassana-insight-meditation/.

Thorp, Tris. "Guided Meditation: Ground Yourself Using the Earth Element." Chopra. February 4, 2019. https://chopra.com/articles/guided-meditation-ground-yourself-using-the-earth-element.

Chapter 5: Tuesday: Engaging the Sacral Chakra on the Day of Joy

Chia, Mantak. *The Inner Smile: Increasing Chi through the Cultivation of Joy*. Rochester, VT: Destiny Books, 2008.

———, and Michael Winn. *Taoist Secrets of Love: Cultivating Male Sexual Energy*. Santa Fe, NM: Aurora Press, 1984.

Clifford, M. Amos. *Your Guide to Forest Bathing: Experience the Healing Power of Nature*. Newburyport, MA: Conari Press, 2018.

Levine, Jessica. "5 Pranayama Techniques with the Power to Transform Your Practice—and Your Life." *Yoga Journal*. Updated February 28, 2018. https://www.yogajournal.com/practice/importance-breath-yoga.

Lindberg, Sara. "How to Do Tai Chi." Healthline. June 3, 2019. https://www.healthline.com/health/exercise-fitness/tai-chi-moves.

Yeshe, Lama. *The Bliss of Inner Fire: Heart Practice of the Six Yogas of Naropa*. Somerville, MA: Wisdom Publications, 1998.

Chapter 6: Wednesday: Engaging the Solar Plexus Chakra on the Day of Power

Abbate, Skya. "The Hara, the Source of Life and the Navel, the Gate of the Spirit." Southwest Acupuncture College. Accessed October 6, 2020. https://acupuncturecollege.edu/blog/hara-source-life-and-navel-gate-spirit.

Aiden, Ashton. "Learn How to Practice Breath of Fire Pranayama in This Quick Tutorial." YogiApproved.com. Accessed October 6, 2020. https://www.yogiapproved.com/om/breath-of-fire-tutorial/.

Gurdjieff and the Fourth Way. "Self-Remembering." Learning Institute for Growth, Healing, and Transformation. http://www.gurdjiefffourthway.org/pdf/SELF-REMEMBERING.pdf.

Hof, Wim. "Guided Wim Hof Method Breathing." YouTube, November 26, 2019. https://www.youtube.com/watch?v=tybOi4hjZFQ.

Kabat-Zinn, Jon. "Mountain Meditation Script." Palouse Mindfulness. Accessed October 5, 2020. https://palousemindfulness.com/docs/mountain meditation.pdf.

Mackay, Jory. "Science Says These 7 Attention Exercises Will Instantly Make You More Focused." *Inc.* September 28, 2017. https://www.inc.com/jory-mackay/sciences-says-these-7 -attention-exercises-will-make-you-more-focused-right -now.html.

Osho. *Meditation: The First and Last Freedom.* New York: St. Martin's Griffin, 2004.

Tubali, Shai, and Tim Ward. *Indestructible You: Building a Self that Can't Be Broken.* London: Changemakers Books, 2015.

Chapter 7: Thursday: Engaging the Heart Chakra on the Day of Love

Anonymous. "How to Practice Compassion Meditation." WikiHow. Last modified September 3, 2020. https://www .wikihow.com/Practice-Compassion-Meditation.

Chödrön, Pema. "How to Practice Tonglen." Lion's Roar. August 26, 2020. https://www.lionsroar.com/how-to-practice -tonglen/.

Embodied Philosophy. "The Six Stages of Metta-Bhavana (Loving Kindness)." Embodied Philosophy. May 17, 2016. https:// www.embodiedphilosophy.com/six-stages-metta-bhavana -loving-kindness/.

Little, Tias. "Awakening the Power of the Heart: Two Sacred Yogic Meditations for Activating and Opening the Heart Chakra." *ConsciousLifestyle.* Accessed September 3, 2020. https://www.consciouslifestylemag.com/heart-chakra -opening-meditation/.

Osho. "The OSHO Mystic Rose Meditation." Osho. Accessed September 3, 2020. https://www.osho.com/highlights-of -oshos-world/mysticrose.

Chapter 8: Friday: Engaging the Throat Chakra on the Day of Expression

Ackerly, Spafford C. "Inner Smile and Healing Sounds." Mantak Chia. Accessed October 6, 2020. https://www.mantakchia .com/inner-smile-and-healing-sounds/.

Ament, Rachel. "Try These Mantras for Anxiety When You're Feeling Overwhelmed." Shape. September 2, 2020. https:// www.shape.com/lifestyle/mind-and-body/mantras-for -anxiety.

O'Brien, Barbara. "Right Speech From the Buddhist Eightfold Path." Learn Religions. Updated January 21, 2019. https:// www.learnreligions.com/right-speech-450072.

Chapter 9: Saturday: Engaging the Third Eye Chakra on the Day of Wisdom

Gaia Staff. "How to Harness the Power of the Shri Yantra." Gaia. November 15, 2019. https://www.gaia.com/article/what-is -the-power-of-shri-yantra.

Godman, David, ed. *Be As You Are: The Teachings of Sri Ramana Maharshi*. London: Penguin, 1985.

Gu, Guo. *Passing Through the Gateless Barrier: Koan Practice for Real Life*. Boulder, CO: Shambhala, 2016.

Katz, Lawrence C., and Manning Rubin. "14 Weird Brain Exercises That Help You Get Smarter." The Healthy. Updated October 18, 2019. https://www.thehealthy.com/aging/mind-memory/brain-exercise/.

Kornfield, Jack. "Audio: A Mind Like Sky Meditation." Jack. Accessed October 5, 2020. https://jackkornfield.com/a-mind-like-sky/.

Venkatesananda, Swami, trans. *The Supreme Yoga: Yoga Vasistha*. Delhi: Motilal Banarsidass Publishers, 2010.

Watson, Rita. "Three Ways to Rewrite Your Story and Embrace the Future." *Psychology Today*. June 15, 2012. https://www.psychologytoday.com/us/blog/love-and-gratitude/201206/three-ways-rewrite-your-story-and-embrace-the-future.

Chapter 10: Sunday: Engaging the Crown Chakra on the Day of Spirit

Chia, Mantak. *Awaken Healing Energy through the Tao: The Taoist Secret of Circulating Internal Power*. Santa Fe, NM: Aurora Press, 1983.

Cronkleton, Emily. "What Are the Benefits and Risks of Alternate Nostril Breathing?" Healthline. Updated July 9, 2018. https://www.healthline.com/health/alternate-nostril-breathing.

Harris, Jules Shuzen. "How to Practice Zazen." Lion's Roar. July 28, 2019. https://www.lionsroar.com/how-to-practice-zazen/.

Rosenberg, Larry. "The Supreme Meditation." Lion's Roar. September 15, 2020. https://www.lionsroar.com/the-supreme-meditation/.